ATRIAL FIBRILLATION

HOW A PHYSICIAN CONVERTED HIS ATRIAL FIBRILLATION TO NORMAL HEART RHYTHM WITH A LOW-RISK, LOW-COST PROTOCOL

MY ZEBRA TREATMENT PROTOCOL

Alan A. Wanderer, M.D.

Anson Publishing, LLC
3701 Trakker Trail
Suite 1B
Box 338
Bozeman, MT 59718

© Copyright by Alan A. Wanderer, M.D.

All rights reserved. No part of this book may be used or reproduced and/or transmitted in any form whatsoever by an electronic or mechanical means, including information storage and retrieval systems, without written permission from the publisher, Anson Publishing, LLC, except a reviewer who may quote brief passages in a review.

For information or permission,
email: **aw.afzebra@gmail.com**

ISBN-979-8-218-52742-6

Library of Congress Control Number: 2024916378

First edition: October 2024
Modified version April 2025

Printed in the U.S.A.

DEDICATION

For my two brothers who passed in 2024.

Warren passed from a complication of AF. A special man who experienced adversities with extraordinary grace and fortitude. His example encouraged me never to give up when dealing with hardship and kept me focused on goals like writing this book.

Richard passed from a heart block and a severe heart valve condition. He pursued excellence in many professions as an advertising executive, attorney, and writer. He was always a gentleman, loved by his peers and family, and he, too, kept me focused on being the best I could be.

Disclosure re' conflict of interest:

The author reports no financial relationships with any company or product(s) mentioned in this book that could be construed as a conflict of interest.

Disclaimer for this book:

This publication/book is provided for educational and informational purposes only and does not constitute providing medical advice or professional services. The information provided should not be used for diagnosing or treating a health problem without involving a health care professional ("HCP"). Never disregard professional medical advice or delay in seeking the same because of something you have read in this book by Alan A. Wanderer, M.D. If you think you may have a medical emergency, call 911 or go to the nearest emergency room immediately. No physician-patient relationship is created by this publication/book or by purchase or use of the same. Neither Alan A. Wanderer, M.D. nor Anson Publishing, LLC, nor any of its members, nor any employee, agent, or representative of Alan A. Wanderer M.D. or Anson Publishing, LLC, nor any contributor to this publication/book, makes any representations, expressed or implied, with respect to the information provided herein or to its use or efficacy.

Abbreviations:
AF= atrial fibrillation
SR= sinus rhythm
Mg= magnesium
K= potassium

TABLE OF CONTENTS

INTRODUCTION

CHAPTER ONE: My Zebra Treatment Protocol for AF

CHAPTER TWO: AF its symptoms and treatment options

CHAPTER THREE: Causes of AF

CHAPTER FOUR: Predisposing factors for AF

CHAPTER FIVE: Role of Mg & K in generating normal heart rhythm and rate

CHAPTER SIX: Evidence Mg and/or K deficiency is associated with a higher incidence of AF. Conversion of AF to SR with Mg/K supplements

CHAPTER SEVEN: Causes of Mg/K deficiencies and extended incubation time required to replenish Mg deficiency

CHAPTER EIGHT: Replenishing Mg deficiency with supplements and foods

CHAPTER NINE: Markers (tests) that may indicate Mg supplementation can convert AF to SR (Fig.1) and reflect a beneficial effect on the heart.

CHAPTER TEN: Replenishing K deficiency with supplements and foods

CHAPTER ELEVEN: The importance of maintaining hydration to avoid triggering AF

CHAPTER TWELVE: The importance of frequent EKG monitoring

CHAPTER THIRTEEN: Graph of my results (Fig.2) demonstrating conversion of AF to SR with My Zebra Treatment Protocol

CHAPTER FOURTEEN: Outline of My Zebra Treatment Protocol and its associated risks.

CHAPTER FIFTEEN: Key points I learned from implementing My Zebra Treatment Protocol

CHAPTER SIXTEEN: A unified theory explaining why inflammation and Mg deficiency cause AF; the involvement of an uncontrolled immune mechanism causing the inflammation; how unhealthy lifestyles stimulate this immune mechanism; and why replenishing Mg may reverse AF to SR.

CHAPTER SEVENTEEN: Final comments

APPENDIX ONE:	Medical consequences associated with AF interventions
APPENDIX TWO:	Recommended daily allowance (RDA) for elemental Mg
APPENDIX THREE:	Foods with high Mg content
APPENDIX FOUR:	Chart for Mg/K supplements
APPENDIX FIVE:	Foods with high K content

BIBLIOGRAPHY

ACKNOWLEDGEMENTS

Abbreviations:
AF= atrial fibrillation
SR= sinus rhythm
Mg= magnesium
K= potassium
HCP= health care professional
RDA= recommended daily allowance

INTRODUCTION:

This book describes my experience with AF. I coined a new word, "auto-cardiography," to describe my heart history, specifically a low-risk, low-cost protocol that converted my AF to SR (normal heart rhythm). I am not a cardiologist or an integrative physician, despite developing a protocol that includes Mg and K supplements. I am board-certified in clinical immunology and allergy with a foundation in clinical and scientific medical research. My medical education included internal medicine, which provided me with basic training in cardiology and the ability to interpret common EKG abnormalities. 'My Zebra Treatment Protocol,' which is explained in the next chapter, describes 25 months of self-observation and treatment. Asymptomatic AF was documented by a Holter monitor, indicating it occurred 39% of the time over 7 days. I unexpectedly converted my AF to SR while on oral Mg supplements, observed by continuous self-monitoring of my EKGs 3-4 times daily. SR occurred 24 weeks after starting the Mg supplements, and I have remained in SR for 19 months to date. I experienced five transient breakthroughs, two due to dehydration, of which one was associated with acute bronchitis and fever, two after I reduced my Mg dose, and one related to K deficiency caused by a diuretic. All reversed to SR when I addressed the causes. The AF breakthroughs indicated my protocol was not a cure but a means to control it. Consequently, my protocol emphasizes the importance of Mg, K, hydration, daily EKG monitoring, and adding foods fortified in Mg and K. Mg and K supplements alone did not meet my daily RDA for both.

My conversion from AF to SR took 24 weeks, which is supported by underappreciated scientific observations discussed in the book. Waiting 24 weeks would not be appropriate if an HCP recommends an immediate therapeutic intervention. I was on an anticoagulant and didn't require an intervention. However, even on an anti-coagulant, cardiology guidelines indicate if one is experiencing AF, the risk of stroke is lessened, but it still exists. Medical literature suggests by converting to SR, I reduced my risk of stroke, but not to the level if I had never experienced AF.

Mg supplementation for AF has been controversial despite three long-term observational studies (two for 20 years and one for 2 years) demonstrating a strong correlation between a high incidence of AF and low blood Mg levels (**CHAPTER SIX** for details). Another study described in the same chapter reported 35 % of post-menopausal women on a strict low Mg diet developed AF and other arrhythmias.

Three studies designed to determine if oral Mg supplementation would benefit AF (**CHAPTER EIGHT**) produced inconsistent results. The designs of the studies were flawed because the Mg supplements (Mg oxide, Mg hydroxide, and Mg sulfate) have poor absorption; two were administered for short durations, and daily EKG monitoring was not part of the protocols. As a result, cardiology has bypassed oral Mg supplementation as a potential option for controlling AF. In essence, there is a need for carefully designed double-blind studies for AF with a protocol that includes oral Mg supplements with good absorption (**CHAPTER EIGHT**), are administered for extended durations (at least 20 to 30 weeks, includes daily EKG monitoring and emphasizes maintaining hydration and addition of foods fortified in Mg and K. I believe until that occurs, the at-large AF community will depend on unscientific claims by Mg manufacturers and the benefit of oral Mg supplementation will remain anecdotal and controversial.

My protocol may only be effective for me. Anyone considering its implementation should have their medical history reviewed by a healthcare professional (HCP) to confirm it is suitable for them. Mg can lower heart rate and/or blood pressure. Someone with pre-existing low blood pressure or a slow heart rate (bradycardia), Mg may cause dizziness or even fainting. It can also cause muscle weakness. The protocol lists other exclusions for candidacy, such as chronic kidney disease and concomitant severe heart disease determined by a cardiologist or other HCP.

Based on my auto-cardiography, this protocol may have potential applications for some individuals with AF. There is no assurance it will be beneficial without randomized controlled trials. However, if determined efficacious, it may prevent recurring paroxysmal AF, persistent or long-standing persistent AF, recurrences of AF after interventions such as cardiac ablation or electrical cardioversion, and AF following cardiac surgery. Assuming the above indications are proven efficacious, it would provide a low-risk option for individuals with AF deemed suitable candidates for this protocol. **All of the above require HCP approval and supervision.**

My clinical research focused on inflammatory mechanisms associated with a genetic disorder characterized by cold-induced acute inflammation. I collaborated with a clinical immunologist/allergist, Dr. Hal Hoffman, who discovered the mutated gene and its protein (called cryopyrin) underlying this condition[1]. Other researchers subsequently recognized this protein is the essential component of a new innate (i.e., born with) immune mechanism which, when out of control, can cause chronic inflammation. It was first named the cryopyrin inflammasome, now referred to as the NLRP-3 inflammasome[1]. I was unaware that activation of the NLRP-3 in the heart could induce chronic inflammation and contribute to the pathogenesis of atrial fibrillation (AF)[2]. Additionally, it has been proven that when NLRP-3 is stimulated, it secretes an inflammatory protein that can interfere with energy production needed to generate SR. Mg is also required for energy production in all cells, including heart cells. Consequently, the pathogenesis of AF may be attributed to chronic inflammation triggered by NLRP-3 activation and an energy deficit in heart cells resulting from the combined effects of NLRP-3 stimulation and Mg deficiency. **CHAPTER SIXTEEN** discusses this concept in more detail.

This book is not meant to provide a comprehensive review of AF. Numerous resources are available to provide a more thorough background, some of which are cited in the bibliography.

Abbreviations:
AF= atrial fibrillation
SR= sinus rhythm
Mg= magnesium
K= potassium
Na= sodium
HCP= health care professional
RDA=recommended daily allowance

CHAPTER ONE: My Zebra Treatment Protocol for AF

What does a zebra have to do with AF? During my medical training, I was taught, 'when you hear hoof beats, think of horses, not zebras.' The presumption was doctors should first consider the most likely diagnosis or treatment and not immediately look 'outside the box' to consider uncommon solutions. A fluke sparked an 'outside the box' epiphany and led me to formulate My Zebra Treatment Protocol, which converted my AF to SR.

My Apple Watch alerted me I was experiencing AF. I decided to review EKGs recorded on my iPhone in the previous two years. Several EKGs revealed evidence of AF, and in retrospect, I ignored them, possibly due to denial they were important. I believe I may also have been experiencing AF on a treadmill. My heart rate would increase abruptly to 130 beats/min and return within a minute or less to my base rate of 80-100 beats/min. I dismissed it as a treadmill sensor error. The alert led to extensive medical and cardiac evaluations confirming I had asymptomatic, long-standing persistent AF (more than one year). According to the *American College of Cardiology, 2023 Practice Guidelines for AF*[3], asymptomatic long-standing persistent AF placed me at increased risk for a stroke and heart failure (the heart cannot pump enough blood into the circulatory system, which causes oxygen depletion in vital organs. My cardiologist started me on an anticoagulant (blood thinner) to prevent a stroke. I read that asymptomatic AF has the potential for progression to symptomatic AF, which is a more concerning clinical category. I familiarized myself with current interventions for converting AF to SR in the event my symptoms became more severe and warranted them. **CHAPTER TWO** and **APPENDIX ONE** discuss intervention options in more detail.

A Holter monitor (a heart monitor taped to the chest to record heart rhythms 24/7) indicated I was experiencing AF thirty-nine percent of the time over seven days. While monitoring EKGs' on my Apple Watch, I would sporadically observe SR. Coincidentally, I had started a laxative that contained Mg hydroxide. I knew Mg was an essential component of many enzymes, one of which is called Na/K ATPase, which is necessary for energy production in all cells. This led to my epiphany. Could the Mg in the laxative explain why my AF was occasionally converting to SR? I switched to different Mg supplements and began experiencing SR more frequently. After trial and error changes to my protocol, the number of days affected with AF per month decreased significantly, described in detail in **CHAPTER THIRTEEN.** An article suggested I reduced my risk for a stroke by converting to SR even with a past history of AF[4]. I purchased the Kardia app from Amazon to monitor my heart rhythm on my iPhone three to four times daily. I continued Mg supplementation, and by 24 weeks, the EKGs revealed I was primarily in SR. Could this inexpensive, low-risk, low-cost mineral supplement convert my AF to SR? A repeat seven-day Holter monitor detected no evidence of AF. I was concerned when I suddenly experienced a recurrence of AF for two days. Another medical article noted diuretics cause excessive urinary excretion of Mg and K. Because I was on a diuretic, my HCP increased my dose of an extended-release K supplement. Within twenty-four hours, AF converted to SR.

Another experience made me question the efficacy of my protocol. I contracted a respiratory infection (bronchitis) with a low-grade fever for a few weeks, and my SR reverted to AF. During my recovery, I read an article[5] emphasizing the importance of hydration in preventing AF. The relationship between dehydration and AF is discussed in **CHAPTER ELEVEN. Almost 10 percent of AF-afflicted individuals are chronically dehydrated, and there is 2.3 times greater risk of an ischemic stroke in individuals with AF and dehydration compared to AF without dehydration**[6]. I was not drinking adequate fluids, and fever worsened my dehydration. I increased my fluid intake and within a few days the AF reverted to SR. Another explanation for the recurrence of AF is bronchitis may have caused systemic inflammation that affected the pacemaker in my heart. Additionally, inflammation of the bronchial airways could limit airflow, leading to a transient reduction in blood oxygenation that might trigger AF[7].

I considered discontinuing the Mg supplementation to determine if my AF would return. However, after a conversation with my cardiologist, I was convinced the risk was too great. The few AF recurrences that reversed to SR convinced me that AF was lurking in the background and my protocol was controlling it. Moreover, an independent data analysis confirmed my observations were statistically significant, as discussed in **CHAPTER THIRTEEN**.

The elements of My Zebra Treatment Protocol that I implemented include (1) recognizing important clinical criteria for its implementation described in **CHAPTER FOURTEEN;** (2) the importance of selecting an optimal oral Mg supplement that met the criteria described in **CHAPTERS EIGHT** and **FOURTEEN**; (3) recognizing the oral Mg supplement had to be administered for a minimum of 6 weeks and potentially for 20 to 30 weeks to determine its efficacy converting AF to SR; (4) adding a potassium supplement as needed; (5) encouraging consumption of foods high in Mg and K content since Mg and K oral supplements would not satisfy my daily RDA for both; (6) recognizing AF is associated with dehydration and required maintaining my hydration; (7) monitoring EKGs 3-4 times daily with apps available on smartphones and

(8) frequent interactions with my HCP while implementing this protocol.

It's been essential to self-monitor my heart rhythm with EKGs to determine if I was experiencing AF or SR. Literature claiming a cure for AF-afflicted individuals does not indicate heart rhythms were monitored daily or even weekly. Consequently, asymptomatic AF may have occurred without an individual's awareness. This also applies to outcomes following conventional therapeutic interventions. Because I experienced AF without symptoms, daily EKG monitoring was critical as I might have been misled believing my AF was under control or even cured. By monitoring my heart rhythm with EKGs 3 to 4 times daily, I became aware I did not cure my AF because I had a few minor recurrences, but I effectively controlled it with My Zebra Treatment Protocol.

Abbreviations:
AF = atrial fibrillation
SR= sinus rhythm
Mg= magnesium
K= potassium
HCP= health care professional

CHAPTER TWO: AF its symptoms and treatment options

AF is defined as an irregular heart rhythm, medically referred to as an arrhythmia. AF rhythms are caused by erratic and disorganized electrical impulses in the heart, resulting in irregular heartbeats. During AF, the heart rate may be irregular and/or rapid (more than 100 beats per minute). It is considered a chronic lifetime condition that may be asymptomatic and progress to severe symptomatology. Based on 2023 statistics from the *American College of Cardiology 2023 Practice Guidelines for AF*[3], it affects approximately five to six million people in the United States and fifty million globally. The incidence is increasing due to an aging population, individuals not addressing predisposing risk factors for AF that include unhealthy lifestyles (**CHAPTER FOUR**), and improved detection. It is projected to increase to thirteen million in the United States by 2030[3].

The *American College of Cardiology 2023 Practice Guidelines for AF* [3] indicates it is associated with increased incidence of the following outcomes: *"a 1.5- to 2-fold increased risk of* **death***; 2.4-fold risk of* **stroke***; 1.5-fold risk of cognitive impairment or* **dementia***; 1.5-fold risk of* **myocardial infarction** *(heart attack); 2-fold risk of* **sudden cardiac death***; 5-fold risk of* **heart failure***; 1.6-fold risk of* **chronic kidney disease***; and 1.3-fold risk of* **peripheral artery disease***.*

In Medicare beneficiaries[3], the most frequent outcome in 5 years after AF diagnosis was **_death_** *(19.5% at 1 year; 48.8% at 5 years;* **_heart failure_** *(13.7%), new-onset **stroke** (7.1%),* **_gastrointestinal hemorrhage_** *(5.7%), and* **_myocardial infarction_** *(3.9%).* AF's association with these serious outcomes has garnered considerable attention from medical and surgical professionals, prompting the development of effective new treatment options.

It is estimated fifty to eighty percent of individuals with AF are initially asymptomatic, referred to as sub-clinical AF. The *American College of Cardiology2023 Practice Guidelines for AF* [3] has defined the following categories for AF:

- Subclinical AF, previously called asymptomatic
- First detected AF: the first documentation of AF regardless of previous symptoms
- Paroxysmal AF: intermittent and originates and terminates within seven days
- Persistent AF: exists for more than seven days up to one year
- Long-standing persistent AF: exists for more than one year
- Permanent AF: when the individual with AF and

the clinician stop further attempts to restore and/or maintain SR

Symptoms associated with AF include:
- Palpitations
- Rapid heart rate
- Dizziness
- Fainting
- Chest pain
- Shortness of breath
- Excessive fatigue and weakness
- Confusion
- Excessive urination caused by production of a diuretic-like protein(i.e. natriuretic peptide) from hearts with AF.

Symptoms associated with AF may occur because of inefficient contraction and propulsion of blood into the arterial circulation. Additionally, excessive urination experienced during AF may lead to excretion of water and sodium, both of which can cause fatigue, weakness, and confusion. Non-specific symptoms such as weakness and fatigue may be attributed to other conditions, which can delay the diagnosis of AF. Paradoxically, there was a greater chance of experiencing a stroke when I was asymptomatic versus having heart palpitations because palpitations may have encouraged earlier medical intervention. Fortunately, my asymptomatic atrial fibrillation (AF) was detected by my Apple Watch, which led to prompt medical evaluation. When diagnosed with asymptomatic AF, even on an anticoagulant, my stroke risk remained higher compared to being in SR[4].

The effectiveness of conventional interventions is less responsive for individuals who have persistent (up to one year) or long-standing persistent (more than one year) duration of AF. Longer duration of AF is associated with continuous chronic inflammation causing changes, such as anatomical remodeling in the heart. These changes may include fibrosis (scarring), enlargement and stretching of heart anatomy, particularly the left atrium, and valve incompetency, which causes backward flow of blood, resulting in heart failure. Several interventions are available to convert AF to SR.

- **Medications** are the most common intervention to control heart rate and rhythm. Many antiarrhythmic agents have a paradoxical risk of causing severe arrhythmias and require close monitoring[3]. Some also have uncomfortable side effects that lead to discontinuation. Recurrences of AF can occur when on these medications. Although they may be permanently effective in converting AF to SR, they are sometimes considered a stopgap for cardiac ablation, as described below.
- **Electrical cardioversion** is another option

which delivers quick, low-energy shocks to the chest. It may be immediately effective, but the conversion is frequently not permanent.

Surgical procedures:

- **Cardiac ablation** is not considered a surgical procedure, but I included it in this category because it may require general anesthesia or deep sedation, and the procedure may last between 1 to 3 hours. The electrophysiologist (EP is a subspecialist in cardiology) threads a catheter through the leg or neck veins into the right upper chamber (right atrium) of the heart, then through the wall (septum) into the left upper chamber (left atrium), where erratic electrical impulses reside. The EP maps the heart for locations of abnormal electrical impulses causing AF. The procedure typically involves the isolation of pulmonary veins (veins that carry oxygenated blood from the lungs to the left atrium), where AF-inducing heart cells are located. Once identified, they are ablated using various techniques, including heat from radiofrequency probes, cold with cryotherapy, laser energy, and pulsed-field ablation (PFA), which involves short bursts of high-voltage electrical energy. Ablation procedures destroy heart tissues which cause the chaotic and irregular electrical impulses. Studies suggest ablation might lower the risk for stroke in some patients with early onset asymptomatic or symptomatic AF, particularly for individuals with a high risk of stroke who are on an anti-coagulant determined by the cardiac acronym CHA2DS2-Vasc[3,4]. It represents the following:

- **C:** Congestive heart failure (1 point)
- **H:** Hypertension (1 point)
- **A2:** Age ≥75 years (2 points)
- **D:** Diabetes mellitus (1 point)
- **S2:** Stroke/TIA/thromboembolism (2 points)
- **V:** Vascular disease (1 point)
- **A:** Age 65-74 years (1 point)
- **Sc:** Sex category (female 1 point)

An individual with AF having a score of 2 or more is considered a candidate for anticoagulation. The higher the number, the greater the risk of stroke.

- **Implantation of a pacemaker with atrioventricular node ablation (AVNA)** to regulate AF is another treatment option. It is considered an option for AF associated with a rapid heart rate and/or rhythm that is refractory to other interventions. It involves radiofrequency (heat generation) ablation or cryotherapy ablation of the atrioventricular (AV) node. The AV node is situated in the right atrium (the upper right chamber) near the junction with the right ventricle (the lower right heart chamber). It transmits electrical impulses from the upper chambers (right and left atrium) to the lower chambers (right and left ventricles), and by eliminating the AV node, rapid or irregular electrical impulses are not relayed to the ventricles. By eliminating the AV node, the implantation of an electronic pacemaker enables control and regulation of electrical impulses, resulting in regular heartbeats. There are pacemakers with leads attached to the heart and also leadless electronic pacemakers.

- **Catheter procedures called**

"transcatheter endovascular left appendage closure" (LAAC) can seal off a pouch (appendage) in the left atrium that may contain blood clots, thereby reducing the risk of a stroke. It is sometimes referred to as the Watchman, referring to a specific device used for this procedure. When installed, conventional anticoagulants may be discontinued, although there is controversy surrounding this decision, which should be made by the HCP. The procedure is considered low-risk but has occasional serious consequences.

- **The Cox-maze IV** procedure is a more invasive open-heart procedure involving precise incisions in the upper heart chambers (atria) that create maze-like scar tissue to block the abnormal electrical circuits causing AF. The cardiac surgeon may also remove or close off the small appendage of the left atrium where clots typically form, thereby reducing the risk of dislodging clots that can cause strokes.

- **A less invasive maze procedure, sometimes called the Wolf mini-maze procedure,** uses a thoracoscope (a tube) with a small camera on the end. A small incision is made between the ribs, and the thoracoscope is inserted with other instruments to ablate the tissues causing AF.
- **Convergent therapy** refers to a hybrid procedure that combines ablation inside the heart by an EP and minimally invasive cardiac surgery on the outside of the heart, involving thoracoscopy.. Both target heart

tissues generating AF. It is considered for AF-afflicted individuals with persistent or long-standing persistent AF, especially if they have failed other interventions.

APPENDIX ONE details the rare but significant medical consequences associated with these interventions. It also lists their AF recurrence rates.

These interventions would be indicated for my AF if recommended by my HCP to control symptoms, such as rapid heart rate, heart failure, concerns about a clot in my heart, or other medical indications. Since those concerns were not present, as long as I maintained SR, I elected to continue my low-risk, low-cost protocol.

Abbreviations:
AF= atrial fibrillation
AFL= atrial flutter
SR= sinus rhythm
PVCs= premature ventricular contractions
Mg= magnesium
K= potassium
HCP= health care professional
EKG= electrocardiogram

CHAPTER THREE: Causes of AF

The heart is an incredibly efficient pump that produces a regular heartbeat, viewed on an EKG as SR. It comprises four chambers: the right upper atrium, the right lower ventricle, the left upper atrium, and the left lower ventricle. Blood lacking oxygen flows from veins into the right atrium, then into the right ventricle. Unoxygenated blood then flows from the pulmonary arteries to the lungs to receive oxygen. Blood that is oxygenated enters the left atrium through the pulmonary veins, flows into the left ventricle, and is finally distributed throughout the arterial circulation.

The electrical impulses in the heart emanate from specialized heart cells in the right atrium. These heart cells are commonly referred to as the pacemaker, anatomically known as the sinoatrial node. The pacemaker cells can automatically generate electrical activity. The electrical activity in the heart is hierarchal. It originates at the top of the heart, in the right atrium, and spreads across both atria, causing them to contract and pump blood into the ventricles. The electrical impulses then flow to the heart's center, the atrioventricular node, where heart cells act as gatekeepers, imperceptibly slowing the electrical impulses to allow the atria time to completely empty their blood into the ventricles. Electrical impulses spread to the ventricles, stimulating them to contract and pump venous blood from the right ventricle to the lungs and oxygenated blood from the left ventricle into the arterial circulation. When the heart is in AF, irregular electrical impulses from the left atrium prevent the atria from contracting efficiently and emptying blood entirely into the ventricles. One of the causes of heart failure associated with AF is blood is inadequately pumped into the arterial circulation and consequently backs up causing fluid to accumulate in the lungs and the extremities. The blood remaining in the left atrium can stagnate to form clots that can dislodge and travel to the brain, creating the risk of strokes.

As mentioned, the heart's electrical signal is hierarchal. When the pacemaker stops functioning in the right atrium, other heart cells take over in the left atrium, located around the base of the pulmonary veins. They produce electrical impulses that cause chaotic, irregular heart rhythms recognized as AF. If those heart cells fail, heart cells in the middle of the heart generate electrical impulses that cause contractions. This abnormal origin of electrical impulses can be treated with a pacemaker, an electronic device installed under the skin with wire leads attached to the heart to create an on-demand electrical pacemaker. On occasion, the electrical signal can initiate in either ventricle. The resulting abnormal heartbeats, called PVCs, can occur with AF and are common with aging. They do not require medical intervention for less than five to six per minute. However, if they become more frequent, they may lead to intervention to prevent life-threatening arrhythmias.

Why would the pacemaker stop generating SR? Heart cells can become thickened and fibrotic (scarred) with calcifications and anatomical remodeling (changes in anatomical structure), rendering them non-functional and altering normal electrical pathways. The reason for this pathology is uncertain, although researchers now consider it may be due to unchecked chronic inflammation. In the **INTRODUCTION and CHAPTER SIXTEEN**, I mentioned the potential role of the NLRP-3 inflammasome causing chronic inflammation in the heart, resulting in AF. Other factors predisposing to AF are listed in **CHAPTER FOUR.**

Does the pacemaker fade away and stop working? The answer is neither yes or no because SR conversion by interventions can be effective for some, but not all AF-afflicted individuals. Interventional treatments attempting to convert AF to SR are more effective if AF is experienced for shorter durations of less than a year. AF of longer duration can be resistant to conversion because pathological and electrical remodeling of the heart may adversely affect the pacemaker.

Two other abnormal heart rhythms originate in the upper chambers (atria). One rhythm similar to AF is atrial flutter (AFL). It originates in the right atrium and occasionally in the left atrium. It is characterized by circular electrical impulses that cause rapid, regular heartbeats of 100 to 150 per minute. It may cause many of the same medical consequences affecting AF, including increased risk of strokes. Treatment is similar to AF and includes anticoagulants, anti-arrhythmic medications, electric cardioversion, and catheter ablation. Another abnormal atrial heart rhythm, called atrial tachycardia, can also originate in the upper chambers of the heart (atria). It is characterized by a rapid heartbeat (150 beats per minute) and causes symptoms such as palpitations, dizziness, and shortness of breath. It may be associated with anatomical defects in the heart, high blood pressure, overactive thyroid, stress, and excessive caffeine or alcohol. The treatment may be similar to AF. Both abnormal heart rhythms can be diagnosed and differentiated by EKGs.

The following chapter identifies predisposing factors that can trigger and/or cause AF.

Abbreviations
AF= atrial fibrillation
Mg = magnesium
K = potassium
Na= sodium
SR= sinus rhythm
HCP = healthcare professional

CHAPTER FOUR: Predisposing factors for AF

This chapter outlines factors that may cause or predispose one to develop AF. I tried to minimize my risk of AF recurrences by adopting a healthier lifestyle. There are risk factors I could not alter, such as inheriting genes from my family with a history of AF, my age as the risk for AF increases as I get older, or my European ancestry. Lifestyles I could change included avoiding artificial sweeteners, improving my diet by avoiding processed foods, maintaining a healthy weight, reducing stress, being more physically active, and limiting my alcohol intake to one or two drinks of wine or beer per week. As detailed in **CHAPTER ELEVEN**, I learned dehydration can significantly cause AF, so maintaining hydration was very important. My other risk factor was sleep apnea, which I addressed with a sleep study and CPAP treatment ten years before I developed AF.

A theme worthy of brief discussion is the role of inflammation as a cause or trigger of atrial fibrillation (AF). I briefly mentioned the involvement of a specific immunity mechanism in **CHAPTER ONE** that can cause dysregulated, out-of-control inflammation that may be an underlying cause of AF. It is called the NLRP 3 inflammasome and is discussed in **CHAPTER SIXTEEN**. Known triggers of the NLRP-3 are listed in red. Some can be minimized by making healthier lifestyle changes.

Risk Factors and medical conditions that increase the prevalence of AF, see references[3,49]

- European ancestry, Caucasian; women more than men
- Elderly because of aging of the heart
- Hereditary history: DNA analysis may reveal genes of which there are approximately one hundred associated with propensity to develop AF
- **Smoking**
- Sedentary lifestyle
- Dehydration
- Excessive endurance exercising (marathons) > 50 years of age
- Pregnancy
- **Excessive alcohol**
- Caffeine
- Eliminate processed foods that are low in Mg and K
- **Type 1 and 2 diabetes mellitus**. Fifteen percent of people with diabetes mellitus have AF, and thirty percent of AF cases occur in diabetics
- **Obesity**
- **COPD (chronic obstructive pulmonary**

disease)
- **Gout**
- Stress
- **Sleep disturbance and sleep apnea**
- Cardiac conditions: heart failure; history of heart attacks (myocardial infarctions); other arrhythmias such as atrial flutter; angina (chest pain caused by not receiving enough oxygen-rich blood to the heart); coronary artery disease; valve disorders (mitral valve and others); pericarditis (infection of sac surrounding the heart; myocarditis (infection in heart cells); **elevated cholesterol causing atherosclerosis (thickening of blood vessels by cholesterol deposits)**; hypertension; during or after cardiac surgery; frequent premature atrial contractions (PACs)
- Chronic kidney disease
- **Chronic inflammatory bowel diseases** may interfere with absorption of Mg and K
- **Infections:** sepsis (pathogens in blood circulation); covid; other pathogens can cause

onset of AF;

- Hyperthyroidism (increased thyroid hormone activity)
- Exposure to high air pollution
- Medication interactions with Mg (I routinely check medications on reliable internet resources to determine if they interact with Mg)
    o Proton pump inhibitors for gastritis and ulcers (Prevacid;®, Nexium®) can alkalinize small intestinal fluids and reduce the absorption of Mg supplements;
    o Some antibiotics: Vibramycin (doxycycline) and Cipro (ciprofloxacin) can decrease Mg absorption;
    o Cancer chemotherapy medications may interfere in the absorption of Mg;
    o Mg can decrease absorption of bisphosphonates to treat and prevent

osteoporosis, such as Fosamax (alendronate) and Boniva (ibandronate)
- Diuretics (furosemide and chlorothiazide) can cause deficiency of Mg and K due to excess urinary excretion;
- Combination of beta-blockers (e.g., atenolol, propranolol) and Mg supplements can lower heart rate, blood pressure, and potentially cause dizziness and fainting; Mg supplements containing zinc and/or calcium can interfere in Mg absorption.

- <u>Medications and supplements that can cause or induce AF.</u> I make an effort to check my medications on the internet to be sure they do not increase risk of AF and not interfere with absorption of Mg.
  - Artificial sugar substitutes in beverages, especially containing aspartame and excess

sugar-sweetened beverages (sucrose, high fructose corn syrup, or fruit juice concentrates). A study indicated individuals drinking artificially sweetened beverages or sugar-sweetened beverages of >2 L/week had a 20 percent increased risk for AF. **This equates to drinking six 10-ounce cans of either beverage per week**[19].

- NSAIDS: non-steroid anti-inflammatory drugs such as ibuprofen can be associated with hypertension, heart failure, and AF. They may interact with anti-coagulants and potentially increase the risk of bleeding.
- Steroids (prednisone) doses as low as 7.5 mg a day can increase AF six-fold as they can cause electrolyte changes with retention of Na and loss of K. The Na can lead to fluid retention, resulting in hypertension and heart

failure. K loss can cause AF[20], **CHAPTER SIX.**

- Excessive use of bronchodilator inhalers (albuterol) for asthma and stimulants, pseudoephedrine (Sudafed®) can stimulate the heart and trigger AF.

- Diuretics, such as hydrochlorothiazide and furosemide (Lasix®), can cause loss of Mg and K through urinary excretion and trigger AF.

- Marijuana THC has been associated with raising heart rate and increasing the risk for AF.

- Low doses of vitamin D can increase the risk for AF.

Abbreviations:
AF= atrial fibrillation
SR= sinus rhythm
Mg= magnesium
K= potassium
Sodium= Na
Calcium= Ca
HCP= health care professional

CHAPTER FIVE: Role of Mg & K generating normal heart rhythm and rate.

First, it is necessary to discuss the specialization of heart cells. Some heart cells produce electrical impulses, while others receive and delay the progression of electrical impulses. Others receive electrical impulses, causing them to contract and pump blood into the circulatory system. The heart requires four electrolytes (Na, K, Mg, and Ca) to initiate and conduct electrical impulses. The movement of electrolytes requires energy derived from a readily available molecule, ATP, which stores energy. Enzymes (Na/K ATPase) enhance ATP breakdown (hydrolysis), releasing heat and chemical energy needed for metabolic processes. **ATP and ATPase enzymes require Mg for optimal energy production for heart cells to function efficiently.** When Mg combines with ATP, it changes the ATP molecular structure, which allows ATPase to attach to ATP and break it down to release energy. Energy production fuels electrolyte pumps in heart cells, which are necessary for transporting electrolytes in and out of cell membranes, creating electrical impulses. Without adequate energy, electrolyte (Na, K, Mg, Ca) transport in heart cells is curtailed, which can cause the pacemaker to fail, facilitating heart cells in the left atrium to take over and create non-synchronized, chaotic electrical impulses identified as AF.

Na is involved in electrical impulse generation and maintains water volume/pressure inside cells to prevent them from dehydrating. Ca is involved in the contraction of heart cells, culminating in heartbeats. K is an essential mineral that must be maintained in critical concentrations inside heart cells, allowing pacemaker heart cells to rest before discharging sequential electrical impulses. Low K levels correlate with an increased risk for AF[9], described in detail in **CHAPTER SIX**. If K deficiency exists, Mg may also be deficient. This has been documented[10] in AF-afflicted individuals with low K blood levels whose replenishment with K cannot occur unless Mg is added. A possible explanation for this concurrence is if Mg levels are low, heart cell energy production needed to maintain K inside the cells will decrease. Consequently, K may leak out of heart cells into the blood circulation and then be excreted by the kidneys. Additionally, low Mg levels will reduce the reabsorption of K in the kidneys, resulting in more K being excreted in the urine. Eventually, low blood K levels will increase the risk for AF.

The importance of K in regulating heart rhythm cannot be overstated. I recognized its importance when I experienced a transient recurrence of AF while on a diuretic, which can cause loss of Mg and K through kidney excretion. The AF converted to SR when I increased a prescribed long-acting, slow-release K supplement.

I purposely simplified the process by which electrolytes create electrical impulses in heart cells. A more in-depth discussion of cell electrophysiology is necessary to explain the generation of electrical impulses in the heart.

Normally, before the electrical impulse occurs, the outside of the cell is positive, and the inside is negative, creating a resting membrane (cell wall) potential (voltage differential).This occurs as follows: Sodium a positive ion ($Na+$) and calcium ($Ca++$) are extracellular (located outside the cell wall), maintaining a positive charge on the outside of the cell compared to the negative charge inside the cell. Potassium is a positive ion (K+). It is primarily intracellular (located inside the cell), and despite its positive charge, it is associated with a net negative intracellular charge. Electrolyte pumps dependent on energy maintain Na+ and Ca++ outside the cell membrane and K+ inside the cell.

When an electrical stimulus arrives from pacemaker cells located in the sino-atrial node or from cells preceding another cell in the electrical conduction pathway, heart cells depolarize, and a voltage change occurs, resulting in an electrical impulse. This occurs when Na+ and Ca++ flow inside heart cells, and K+ flows out of cells, making the inside of the cell more positive and the outside more negatively charged. This change in electrical charge creates an electrical impulse that stimulates the contraction of heart cells. When depolarization occurs, Ca++ is involved in the plateau phase of the action potential, prolonging the heart cell contraction.

Mg-containing ATP is catalyzed by enzymes (ATPase), which break down ATP to release energy for electrolyte pumps that control the movement of electrolytes in heart cells. The Na+/K+ pump and Ca++ pump drive Na+ and Ca++ out of the cell and K+ into the cell, creating a new resting membrane potential (voltage differential) with the inside of the heart cell negatively charged and outside positively charged. The cell is now ready for depolarization by electrical impulses from the pacemaker or other cells in the electrical conduction pathway.

It's worth noting that pacemaker cells in the sino-atrial node are specialized to produce automatic electrical impulses. They have an unstable resting membrane potential that spontaneously depolarizes after each action potential. The same electrolytes (Na+, K+, and Ca++) are still involved via different mechanisms, allowing for its automaticity.

Abbreviations:

AF= atrial fibrillation
SR= sinus rhythm
AFL=atrial flutter
PVCs= premature ventricular contractions
Mg= magnesium
K= potassium
HCP= health care professional
EKG= electrocardiogram

CHAPTER SIX: Evidence Mg and /or K deficiency is associated with a higher incidence of AF. Conversion of AF to SR with Mg/K supplements

The following studies provide compelling evidence for the correlation between Mg and/or K deficiency and the predilection for AF. Each article is listed with a summary and a detailed description.

> **Summary** [11]: The Framingham Heart Study observed residents of Framingham, Massachusetts for twenty years to evaluate the epidemiology of heart disease. Researchers concluded there was a higher

prevalence of AF in individuals with the lowest Mg blood levels.

Detailed description: The study included 3530 participants without history or physical evidence of pre-existing cardiovascular disease. They underwent periodic cardiac evaluations over a twenty-year period, and among the 3520 participants, 228 developed atrial fibrillation (AF). Within this group of AF, eighty participants (35%) had the lowest serum Mg levels, suggesting a positive correlation between low serum Mg levels and the development of AF. Subjects with the lowest Mg levels had a fifty percent increased risk for AF compared to participants with Mg levels in the upper limit.

Summary[12]: Postmenopausal women without evidence of preexisting cardiovascular disease or arrhythmias (AF, AFL) were observed in a research unit while on a low Mg diet for seventy-eight days. Five of the fourteen women developed arrhythmias (AF and AFL), which reversed with Mg supplements.

Detailed description: The study involved fourteen post-menopausal women fed a Mg-restricted diet (thirty-three percent of the recommended daily allowance) for seventy-eight days. The participants resided in a research unit for the entire study to carefully monitor their Mg intake. During the low Mg diet phase, heart rhythm abnormalities appeared in five women: two developed AF in combination with AFL, one had AFL and

PVCs, two had PVCs, and one developed a heart block. The AF and AFL reversed to SR with Mg supplementation. The participants with PVCs and heart block took longer to reverse with Mg supplements.

Summary[13]: Individuals with the lowest serum Mg levels had the highest risk for developing AF.

Detailed description: 2228 participants without prior cardiovascular disease were followed over two years, and 162 developed AF. The data indicated a significant correlation between participants with the lowest serum Mg levels and increased incidence of AF.

Summary[14]: The study identified a correlation between low serum Mg and a higher risk for AF. The risk was the same for Caucasians and African Americans.

Detailed description: 14,390 participants free of AF were studied over twenty years. AF was identified in 1,776 participants. They were divided into five groups depending on their serum Mg levels. The highest incidence of AF occurred in participants with the lowest serum Mg levels. The lowest incidence of AF occurred in individuals with average or higher Mg levels. Participants on diuretics also demonstrated a correlation between the lowest Mg levels and a higher risk for AF.

Summary[9]: In this study, low serum levels of K were associated with a higher incidence of AF.

Detailed discussion: The study population consisted of 4059 participants without AF. Over approximately twelve years, 474 developed AF. Low serum K levels were significantly correlated with a higher incidence of AF. Results were independent of age, sex, serum Mg levels, and other medically related variables.

Summary[15]: The study involved electrical cardioversion and observed that administering intravenous solutions of Mg and K improved the success rate converting AF to SR.

Detailed description: Electrical cardioversion was performed on 170 patients with persistent AF. Half the patients received intravenous solutions containing Mg and K during electrical cardioversion; the other half received a placebo. The group that received Mg/K had a significantly higher success rate converting AF to SR compared to the placebo group. Additionally, the Mg/K group required less electrical energy to convert to SR than the placebo group.

The following studies indicate AF-afflicted individuals can have Mg deficiency in their heart cells concomitant with normal serum Mg levels. The determination of Mg deficiency in heart cells of AF individuals was measured by the EXA test. The test relies on data indicating a 100 percent

correlation between the Mg concentration in heart cells (obtained from biopsies of heart tissue during cardiac surgery) and sublingual cells (obtained by scraping cells under the tongue). The test involves X-rays measuring the energy emitted when cells are exposed to X-rays. This test is unfortunately no longer available.

> **Summary**[16]: Twenty-two AF patients undergoing catheter ablation received intravenous Mg sulfate or placebo. All patients had normal baseline serum Mg levels, and 89 percent had a deficiency of Mg in their heart cells. Mg sulfate post-infusion increased serum levels over 6 hours, and Mg levels inside heart cells improved at the 6-hour post-infusion mark.

Detailed description: This double-blind study involved 22 AF participants who received intravenous Mg sulfate or placebo during cardiac ablation. All patients had normal serum Mg levels at baseline, and 89 percent had low Mg concentrations in their heart cells. **These results indicate AF-afflicted individuals can have a normal Mg serum level concomitantly with Mg deficiency in their heart cells.** The intravenous Mg sulfate increased the Mg inside heart cells only at six hours post-infusion.

Summary[17]: Patients on anti-arrhythmic medications had deficiencies of Mg concentrations inside their heart cells. These medications are associated with a potential risk for fatal arrhythmias because they can prolong the EKG QTc interval. The QTc interval measures the time for the ventricles to contract and relax. If it is too long, electrical impulses from the right atrium are delayed, allowing life-threatening ventricular arrhythmias to occur. Treatment with a long-acting oral Mg supplement reduced the risk of fatal arrhythmias by shortening the QTc interval.

Detailed description: 63 percent of patients receiving anti-arrhythmic medications (sotalol or dofetilide) for arrhythmias (AF is assumed as the article didn't specify the type of abnormal rhythms) had low Mg concentrations inside their heart cells. The Mg deficiency in heart cells was corrected within 51 hours with a slow-release oral Mg supplement (Mag-Tab SR, Mg Lactate), and the QTc interval decreased within 3 TO 51 hours post-administration, thereby reducing the risk of fatal arrhythmias. **My comment:** This Mg formulation could be significant for AF conversion because data demonstrated a rapid onset of action of 3 to 51 hours to reduce the QTc and simultaneously normalize Mg concentrations in heart cells. It suggests the incubation period required to achieve an effective blood concentration of Mg with this formulation may be shorter than anticipated with commonly available formulations of oral Mg supplements (discussed in **CHAPTER EIGHT**). Data from the company manufacturing this product supports this observation[18].

Conclusion: Correlation does not always imply causality; consequently, significant medical literature indicates that Mg supplementation for AF conversion to SR is inconclusive. An editorial[19] titled *"Magnesium for AF, Myth or Magic?"* concluded that intravenous Mg sulfate supplementation was inconsistent converting or preventing AF. The reason for this inconsistency may be the half-life of intravenous Mg sulfate used to treat AF is 12 hours and is administered only for a few days[8]. The editorial does not discuss the extended half-life of Mg, which is 6 weeks[22], and that an extended incubation time (possibly 20 to 30 weeks) is likely required to replenish Mg inside heart cells that may convert AF to SR, **CHAPTER SEVEN.**

Abbreviations:
AF= atrial fibrillation
SR= sinus rhythm
Mg= magnesium
K= potassium
RDA=recommended daily allowance

CHAPTER SEVEN: Causes of Mg/K deficiencies and extended incubation time required to replenish Mg deficiency

Estimates in the US indicate between 30 to 50 percent of the population do not consume their RDA of Mg because Western diets contain low Mg content in processed foods. Refining wheat to flour, rice to polished rice, and corn to starch causes an 80 t0 90 percent loss of Mg[20]. Refined salt and drinking soft water also reduce Mg intake. In essence, food technology predisposes populations to an inadequate intake of Mg.

Is there a test to determine if Mg deficiency exists? The standard approach is to obtain serum

Mg levels. **An overlooked observation is the blood compartment represents only one percent of the total body Mg stores[20]. This has major clinical significance because a normal serum Mg will not reflect low Mg concentrations in the heart cells of individuals with AF.** [16,17] Heart cells in the pacemaker and the middle of the heart may not function efficiently if Mg concentrations inside heart cells are low. The electrical impulses from the pacemaker heart cells may fail, and consequently, erratic, chaotic electrical impulses may take over in the left atrium. Additionally, if heart cells in the middle of the heart fail as gatekeepers delaying the progression of electrical impulses into the ventricles, then erratic rapid electrical impulses from the left atrium will be transmitted without delay, causing a fast, irregular heart rate that can result in AF[3].

Can low intracellular Mg concentrations be replenished? This is a controversial question. If it can be replenished, AF may convert to SR or even prophylactically prevent AF recurrences after conventional interventions. One study[12] demonstrated a low Mg diet in post-menopausal women can induce arrhythmias, including AF, which were reversed to SR with oral Mg supplementation. How long does it take to replenish Mg? Studies have shown replenishing Mg stores occurs slowly over many weeks or months. One scientific term worth understanding is *half-life*, which is the time it takes for the amount of a substance in the body to be reduced by one-half. **The half-life of Mg is approximately six weeks**[22]. The amount of Mg stored in humans is excreted by one-half every six weeks. Once Mg is absorbed, it is distributed and exchanged slowly between several anatomical compartments: blood, bones, muscles, and tissues. Assuming there is no pre-existing deficiency of Mg in the body, if Mg was not consumed for 6 weeks, it would require six weeks for administration of elemental Mg to re-establish Mg body stores. Pre-existing Mg deficiency in large populations and AF-afflicted individuals may require several half-lives of Mg to replenish and maintain Mg stores. One study[25] cited in detail below, indicated at least 20 to 30 weeks were required to achieve a steady state of maximum serum Mg concentrations even in healthy subjects treated with oral Mg supplements.

The following articles provide evidence that an extended incubation is needed to replenish Mg stores in humans with oral Mg supplements.

- Article[24] was designed to determine if Mg supplements could benefit individuals with Type 2 diabetes mellitus. The answer was inconclusive, but data indicated Mg supplements required 1 to 3 months to increase and maintain blood Mg levels.

- Based on conclusions in another study[25], at least 20 to 30 weeks were required to achieve a steady state of maximum serum Mg concentrations even in healthy subjects treated with oral Mg supplements containing 300 to 400 mg of elemental Mg per day. A steady state means that the maximum concentration of Mg in the body remains relatively constant. This data is consistent with the extended 6-week half-life of Mg in humans.

- In contrast, another study[17] replenished Mg in heart cells from low to normal concentrations in 3 days. This occurred during treatment with a slow-release oral Mg supplement (Mg L-Lactate as Mag-Tab® SR). This product has excellent absorption of 40 percent and maintains stable Mg serum levels for repeat twenty-four-hour intervals.[17,18] Unfortunately, the study design[17] did not report conversion rates of AF to SR. Nevertheless, it raises the possibility this supplement formulation might require a shorter incubation to convert AF to SR, but more testing is needed to validate this premise.

My conclusion: Significant evidence indicates replenishing Mg deficiency with oral Mg supplementation requires an extended incubation, at least 6 weeks up to a maximum of 20 to 30 weeks.

Future studies are needed to determine if the Mg supplement mentioned in articles[17,18] could convert and maintain AF to SR in a shorter time because of its rapid onset of action, excellent absorption, and ability to maintain blood levels for repeat 24-hour intervals. This Mg supplement has a fast onset of action evidenced by a reduction of the EKG QTc interval within 3 hours and maximized in 51 hours (approximately 2 days) following its administration. The author stated, *"Given the quick onset of appreciable QTc interval reductions with magnesium l-lactate, <u>acute use of the oral product in a patient at risk for TdP (i.e. abnormal heart rhythm) may be possible and would obviate the need for intravenous access.</u>"*

Abbreviations:
AF= atrial fibrillation
SR= sinus rhythm
Mg= magnesium
K= potassium
HCP= health care professional
RDA= recommended daily allowance

CHAPTER EIGHT: Replenishing Mg deficiency with supplements and foods

When Mg concentrations in the body are optimal, there is a balance between the amount absorbed through the intestines and excreted in the urine and stools. As mentioned in **CHAPTER FOUR and SEVEN**, Western diets consist of many processed foods, which cause a deficiency of Mg. Other reasons for Mg deficiency include diuretics, which can cause excessive urinary excretion of Mg, or by not ingesting or absorbing adequate amounts of Mg to maintain Mg balance. **CHAPTER FOUR** lists some medications that can interfere with Mg absorption. In particular, proton pump inhibitors used for treatment of high acidity in the stomach (Nexium®, Prevacid®, etc.) can alkalinize small intestinal fluids, reducing Mg absorption.

Approaches to replenishing Mg include consuming foods high in Mg content, adding supplements containing Mg, or both. The RDA varies depending on sex and age, which is included in **APPENDIX TWO**. Certain foods are known to be high in Mg content (**APPENDIX THREE**). Pumpkin seeds, nuts, halibut, spinach, leafy vegetables, beans, and grains have some of the highest Mg content. Mg supplements and foods fortified with Mg may be needed, especially in AF-afflicted individuals with a high incidence of Mg deficiency in their heart cells. I make a concerted effort to consume foods high in Mg content. Pumpkin seeds are particularly high in Mg content, and I routinely add them to my cereal.

Selecting the best Mg supplement can be daunting when considering the many options in stores or on the internet. Mg supplements are available in many formulations, doses, and combinations of ingredients, making it difficult to make an educated choice. It is an unregulated one-and-one-half billion dollar industry. Labels are often incorrect or deceptive, with unsubstantiated claims and non-standardized doses of elemental Mg per tablet or capsule. Some ethical manufacturers voluntarily go the next step to ensure quality control by manufacturing under *Current Good Manufacturing Practice* guidelines (cGMP), which include third-party audits. The label may include a cGMP logo. I discovered some manufacturers may not list the cGMP label but still conform to quality control. When the label did not list cGMP, I messaged the manufacturer to determine if they complied with that standard before I purchased their product.

Through careful investigation, I learned important facts about Mg supplements.

- **Determining the supplements with the best absorption of Mg**
  - Animal studies[26] tested the absorption of the following Mg supplements: oxide, chloride, sulfate, carbonate, acetate, picolinate, citrate, gluconate, lactate, and aspartate. Organic salts such as gluconate, lactate, and aspartate had better absorption than inorganic salts, like Mg hydroxide and Mg oxide.
  - One study[27] tested Mg supplements in humans and concluded organic Mg supplements, such as Mg lactate and Mg aspartate, are better

absorbed than inorganic salts, except Mg chloride. Mg oxide had very poor absorption.

- Another study[28] compared different Mg supplements, both organic and inorganic and determined organic supplements, namely a long-acting sustained-release Mg L- lactate (Mag-Tab SR®) and Mg aspartate had the best absorption. The least absorbed were Mg hydroxide and Mg carbonate, which are inorganic Mg salts. They have a more significant laxative effect because they are less absorbed and are retained in the intestinal tract.

- A study[29] tested several Mg supplements in humans and were classified according to absorption: excellent (lactate), good (chloride, citrate, fumarate, gluconate, aspartate, and glycinate), and extremely low (oxide). No absorption data was provided for Mg hydroxide, but there was a comment that it is practically insoluble in water, which would imply poor absorption.

Based on these studies, I concluded organic Mg supplements have the best absorption, which equates to more Mg being distributed throughout the body. Filtering all the above data, the following organic Mg supplements had the best absorption: lactate, aspartate, gluconate, glycinate, and citrate. In particular, one organic supplement is well absorbed, Mg L- Lactate Slow Release (Mag-Tab®). The only inorganic Mg supplement with good absorption was Mg chloride. Mg supplements with the least absorption were oxide, carbonate, sulfate, and hydroxide.

APPENDIX FOUR lists organic and inorganic supplements.

- **Determining the percentage of elemental Mg in each dose.**

  o Elemental Mg++ is the form of Mg that is essential for heart cells to function. Calculations are available in **APPENDIX FOUR** to determine the percentage of elemental Mg in supplement doses. **Depending on the Mg supplement, they contain between 7 to 60 % of elemental Mg++. This underscores the need to add foods fortified in Mg (APPENDIX THREE).**

  o Following are examples of why I realized this is important.

    ❖ One label of a Mg gluconate supplement indicated each capsule contained 600 milligrams (mgs) of Mg. It would be incorrect to assume each capsule provided 600 mgs of elemental Mg++. The percentage of elemental Mg++ in the

Mg formulation is seven percent, indicating 600 mgs capsule only contained 42 mgs of elemental Mg^{++}. This is ten percent of the daily recommended amount of elemental Mg^{++} required for an adult male which is approximately 420 mgs. Moreover, only a small percentage of the 42 mgs is absorbed.

❖ The label on a Mg oxide supplement indicated each capsule contains 500 mgs of Mg oxide. It also stated it represents 119 percent of the DV (daily value), which estimates the amount of a specific nutrient needed in a standard daily diet. The DV is broader than the RDA, but both try to estimate the needs for a nutrient. The RDA and DV list the daily amount required for Mg in terms of elemental Mg^{++}. The DV on the label states the Mg oxide in the 500 mg capsule is 119 percent of the DV for Mg, suggesting it supplies more than the RDA of 420 mg of elemental Mg++ for an adult male. However, this implies the 500 mg of Mg oxide is equivalent to elemental Mg++, which is erroneous. The percent of elemental Mg++ in Mg oxide is 60 percent, which in the 500 mg capsule equates to 300 mgs of elemental Mg++. Instead of 119 percent of the DV, the actual number is 71 percent (300 mg /420 mg) for an adult male. The 300 mg of elemental Mg++ per dose is even less meaningful when realizing Mg oxide is poorly absorbed.

- Elemental Mg++ in supplements is not entirely absorbed, and most do not provide the percentage of absorbed Mg. However, previously mentioned studies[18,26-29] provide information that helped me decide which supplements have the best absorption (see earlier comments in this chapter).

- **Side effects of Mg supplements is another consideration**. Almost all Mg supplements have a laxative effect. When Mg supplements have less absorption, Mg will be retained in the intestinal tract and cause more laxative effect. Several studies observed Mg oxide, a popular inorganic Mg supplement, and Mg hydroxide have the most laxative effects. The latter is in Milk of Magnesia ®, a well-known laxative. They may cause diarrhea, resulting in loss of K and water, which can trigger AF.

- **Selecting Mg supplements that can maintain 24-hour blood levels.** Mg stores in Mg-deficient individuals will likely be replenished if consistent blood levels of elemental Mg are maintained over repeat 24-hour intervals.

Supplements with descriptors of sustained-release and slow-release listed on labels may achieve and maintain consistent blood levels of Mg for longer durations. However, that is an assumption unless scientific data supports it, as with Mag-Tab®[18].

- **Avoid Mg supplements that contain extra ingredients**. Zinc[30] and calcium[31] can interfere with Mg absorption. Some supplements include herbs, and others contain several formulations of Mg, which complicates determining the milligram amount of elemental Mg++ in each dose. <u>I only select Mg supplements with a single Mg ingredient and without zinc or calcium.</u>

- **Avoid Mg supplements that list chelation or liposomal descriptors.** Liposomal means the Mg supplement is encased in fat-like particles with the inference it may be better absorbed. The effectiveness of liposomal formulations improving Mg absorption is speculative unless the manufacturer provides scientific data to support their claim. Chelation refers to the attachment of Mg to an organic compound. Organic Mg supplements are all chelated. Listing chelation on a label implies it is a differentiator for better efficacy, suggesting an inaccurate advantage over other Mg supplements.

The following studies were designed to prevent AF with oral Mg supplements. They did not include data determining if the Mg supplements could convert AF to SR.

Summary[32]: Participants for elective heart surgery (coronary artery bypass graft, CABG) received oral Mg sulfate to determine if it reduced the incidence of AF that frequently occurs after the surgical procedure. The Mg sulfate significantly reduced the incidence of AF after surgery compared to placebo.

Detailed description: The participants received oral Mg sulfate or placebo three days before the procedure and on the day of surgery. The Mg sulfate significantly reduced the incidence of AF after surgery.

My comments: This study supports the potential benefit of oral Mg supplementation to prevent AF; however, Mg sulfate was administered for only four days. Long-term administration of Mg sulfate is impractical because it has poor absorption and may cause pronounced gastrointestinal side effects.

Summary[33]: A randomized control trial in an elderly population was performed to assess if oral Mg oxide could reduce the occurrence of premature atrial contractions (PACs) that predispose to developing AF. PACs are extra heartbeats in either upper chambers (left and right atria). There was no difference in the incidence of PACs with Mg oxide or placebo.

Detailed description: 59 elderly (mean age of 62) participants were studied to determine if the incidence of PACs could prophylactically be reduced with Mg oxide. None of the participants had AF. The incidence of PACs was no different between the Mg oxide-treated group and placebo.

My comments: This study did not include individuals with AF, and although PACs can be associated with the development of AF, the incidence of AF was not reported in the study. Long-term administration of Mg oxide is not preferable because it has poor absorption and can cause pronounced gastrointestinal side effects.

Summary[34]: This study was designed to determine if long-term Mg hydroxide versus placebo could decrease the recurrence rate of AF after electrical cardioversion, either alone or in combination with sotalol, an anti-arrhythmic. The results observed over six months revealed no difference in reduction of AF recurrences between Mg hydroxide and placebo groups with or without sotalol.

Detailed description: This study included only patients with a history of persistent AF. Periodic Holter monitoring was used to detect AF. No difference in recurrence of AF was observed following continuous treatment with Mg hydroxide with or without sotalol compared to placebo.

My comments: This study treated patients with Mg hydroxide, one of the least absorbed Mg formulations and the chief component of a commercial laxative, Milk of Magnesia®. Consequently, its poor absorption will reduce its effectiveness reducing recurrences of AF. Monitoring EKGs for AF was not done daily, leaving long gaps when heart rhythm data was not gathered.

My Conclusions: Mg supplements administered in these studies (Mg oxide, Mg hydroxide, and Mg sulfate) have extremely poor absorption, diminishing their therapeutic efficacy. I am unaware of studies designed to convert AF to SR that involved oral Mg supplements with excellent absorption, administered for 20 to 30 weeks, and included daily EKG monitoring.

Abbreviations:
AF= atrial fibrillation
SR= sinus rhythm
Mg= magnesium
K= potassium
Ca= calcium
% HRV= % Heart Rate Variability

CHAPTER NINE: Markers (tests) that may indicate Mg supplementation can convert AF to SR (Fig.1) and reflect a beneficial effect on the heart

CHAPTER SIX established compelling evidence for Mg deficiency in individuals with AF.

CHAPTER SEVEN provided data based on the half-life of Mg in humans in Mg balance is six weeks. The incubation to achieve a steady state of maximum serum Mg concentrations even in healthy humans is at least 20 to 30 weeks[25]. When pre-existing Mg deficiency exists in heart cells of AF-afflicted individuals, administering oral Mg likely will require incubation of several six-week half-lives of Mg, equating to more than six weeks and potentially up to 20 to 30 weeks to achieve a steady state of Mg.

There are no inexpensive readily available markers (tests) that indicate if Mg supplements can improve Mg concentrations in Mg-deficient heart cells of AF-afflicted individuals. One expensive test uses X-ray analysis to determine Mg concentration in sublingual cells obtained by scraping inside an individual's mouth[35]. The results correlated significantly with Mg concentrations in heart cells obtained from heart biopsies. This method has been used in several research studies[16,17] but is unavailable for routine clinical use. The reason for determining Mg concentration in heart cells is if normalization of Mg concentrations occur, it may correlate with the conversion of AF to SR. To date, there are no studies that have determined this correlation.

A marker that may reflect a correlation with the incidence of AF is % **HEART RATE VARIABILITY**(% HRV). It measures the variation in the time interval between consecutive heartbeats in milliseconds (msec). It reflects the autonomic nervous system that controls involuntary bodily functions such as heart rate, blood pressure, digestion, and body temperature. The autonomic nervous system comprises the sympathetic and the parasympathetic nervous systems. The sympathetic nervous system (SNS), commonly called the "fight or flight" response, is activated by stress, which stimulates the release of adrenalin and cortisone compounds. It will increase heart rate, blood pressure, and inhibit digestion, redirecting blood to vital organs (heart and brain). The parasympathetic nervous system (PNS) slows heart rate, reduces blood pressure, stimulates digestion, and promotes relaxation. Conventional thinking is % HRV reflects a balance between the SNS and the PNS. Larger % HRV intervals of 50 to 100 milliseconds suggest a balance between the SNS and PNS and are reflected on graphs as unattenuated or wide variations in millisecond intervals. It appears like a volatile chart of a stock price. If the graph shows attenuated % HRV with small millisecond intervals, it is interpreted as reflecting dominance of the SNS and is associated with more risk for AF. It appears essentially like a flat line chart of a stock price. **Fig. 1** demonstrates the difference between unattenuated and attenuated % HRV.

Some medical conditions can alter the % HRV. These include stress, anxiety, heart disorders like heart failure, coronary artery disease, arrhythmias including AF, diabetes, sleep disorders, and depression. Medications affecting % HRV include beta-blockers that slow heart rate, calcium channel blockers to treat high blood pressure, and some antidepressants. Essentially, medical conditions and medications should remain unchanged to interpret the significance of % HRV. This list is not comprehensive, so I continue to stay abreast of any previously unknown medical conditions or medications that could affect the % HRV.

I was unaware that the HRV was being recorded on my iPhone when I wore my Apple Watch. I plotted this data over 25 months during my treatment with my protocol. During this period, I did not experience new medical conditions or medication changes that could have affected the % HRV. **Fig.2** is a graph of the % HRV, which mirrored the incidence of my AF per month, (**CHAPTER THIRTEEN**). An independent statistical analysis determined a direct correlation between both sets of data, which is discussed in **CHAPTER THIRTEEN.** The % HRV intervals during my outbreaks of AF showed unattenuated (wide millisecond intervals) variability with intervals up to 160 milliseconds between heartbeats. When I had no AF, the % HRV intervals were in the low range of 10 to 20 milliseconds (attenuated), see **Fig.1**. This observation contradicted conventional opinions, as the results suggested the SNS was predominant and controlling my AF. It seemed odd because if that was true, my heart rate and blood pressure should have been elevated, and neither occurred. I considered the % HRV could be a marker for outbreaks of AF. A glance at the graph in **CHAPTER THIRTEEN** shows the correlation between % HRV and the incidence of my AF. **Fig. 1** shows a comparison of unattenuated % HRV in

August 2023 with AF to attenuated % HRV in August 2024 with no AF. **Fig. 2** illustrates this correlation has existed for 25 months.

After reviewing the medical literature, I discovered three articles consistent with my observations. One article[36] reported reviewing Holter monitor readings on 2100 individuals, of whom 782 had hypertension. During a follow-up of approximately one year, 44 individuals developed AF. A higher unattenuated % HRV correlated with occurrences of AF. I don't have hypertension, but it seemed supportive of my observation. Another study[37] reported % HRV may be a prognostic marker for the recurrence of AF after cardiac ablation. All AF-afflicted individuals had unattenuated % HRV preoperatively. Those who continued to have unattenuated % HRV patterns postoperatively eventually had recurrences of AF, and required another catheter ablation. The AF-afflicted individuals who developed post-operative attenuated % HRV did not have recurrences of AF and consequently did not require another catheter ablation. This provided more support for my observation. Animal data is often used to support therapies and medical applications in humans. A study on horses[38] observed % HRV before and after electrical cardioversion for AF. Unattenuated % HRV correlated with the incidence of AF. Conversely, after electrical cardioversion of AF to SR, the HRV was attenuated.

The QTc interval measured on an EKG may be a potential marker for demonstrating a beneficial Mg effect on the heart. The QTc represents the time for the heart's lower chambers (the ventricles) to contract and recover. This measurement is accurate for heart rates between 50 to 100 beats per minute.

The normal QTc for an adult male is 350-450 milliseconds (msec), and 360 to 460 msec for adult women. A long QTc is associated with an increased risk for a ventricular heart rhythm called 'torsades de pointe,' which is a life-threatening arrhythmia. Individuals with Mg deficiency can have prolonged QTc and potentially be at risk for this ventricular life-threatening heart rhythm. Before I started the Mg supplements, my QTc was 484 msec, slightly longer than normal. Several studies demonstrated that administration of Mg intravenously[39,40] or orally[17] can shorten the QTc interval. The observation that Mg reduces the QTc interval indicates it has a beneficial biological effect on heart cells. My QTc gradually decreased on Mg supplementation. My last measurement was 375 msec, a decrease of 22 percent from the QTc measurement before I started Mg supplements. That change may have reduced my risk for the life-threatening arrhythmia and potentially sudden death associated with AF.

The QTc interval can be affected by many medical conditions and medications. Medical conditions that can prolong the QTc interval include inherited disorders, electrolyte imbalances such as low serum concentrations of Mg, Ca, and K, heart failure, coronary artery disease, alcoholism, and infections. Medications that can prolong the QTc interval include but are not limited to antiarrhythmics (amiodarone, sotalol, flecainide, and others); antibiotics (erythromycin, azithromycin, levofloxacin); antihistamines (diphenhydramine, Benadryl ®; cetirizine (Zyrtec®); antidepressants and anti-psychotic drugs; antifungals (ketoconazole); and diuretics such as amiloride (Midamor®). There are medical conditions and medications that can shorten the QTc interval. They include elevated blood levels of K and low thyroid levels. Medicines that can shorten the QTc interval include but are not limited to: beta-blockers, namely atenolol (Tenormin®), propranolol (Inderal ®); calcium channel blockers such as verapamil (Calan®), diltiazem (Cardizem®); and diuretics, such as spironolactone (Aldactone®). These lists are not comprehensive.

Mg supplements can reduce the QTc interval; however, the effect on the heart can only be interpreted if medical conditions and medications remain unchanged after the QTc was first measured. I remain aware of that caution and reliable sources to determine if any new medications or medical conditions could affect the QTc.

I added the QTc in My Zebra Treatment Protocol because a reduction in the QTc by Mg supplements may indicate it has a beneficial effect on my heart. I have followed %HRV and QTc, the former as a marker for recurrence of AF and the latter as a marker indicating a beneficial biological effect of Mg on my heart.

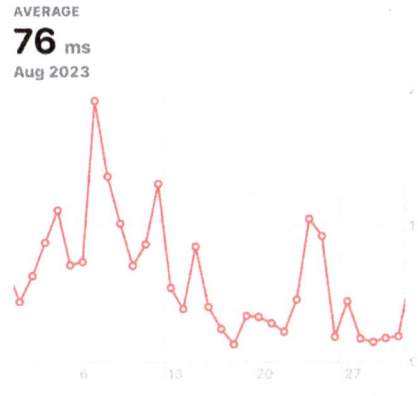

Unattenuated heart rate variability in **August 2023** when I was experiencing AF

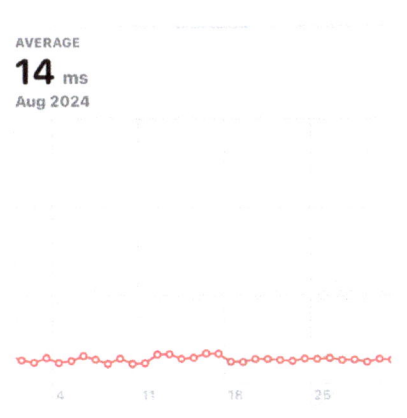

Attenuated heart rate variability in **August 2024** when I had no AF

Fig 1. Examples of unattenuated and attenuated. % heart rate variability (HRV)

Abbreviations
AF= atrial fibrillation
SR= sinus rhythm
Mg= magnesium
K= potassium
KCL= potassium chloride
HCP= health care professional
RDA= recommended daily allowance

CHAPTER TEN: Replenishing K deficiency with supplements and foods.

Chapter SIX describes the study correlating low K blood levels with an increased incidence of AF[9]. K is essential for efficient functioning of heart cells, as described in **CHAPTER FIVE.** Although not well understood, there is recognition that K deficiency frequently occurs with unrecognized Mg deficiency[10], explained in **CHAPTER FIVE.** Consequently, if adding a K supplement doesn't increase K blood levels, there may be a need to increase the Mg supplement to improve K blood levels.

- Although K deficiency is not common, it can occur, especially with diuretics, which may cause excessive excretion by the kidneys. An adequate amount of daily elemental K is between 1600 to 2000 milligrams.

- K supplements are available on the internet and in health food stores. They are listed in **APPENDIX FOUR,** along with the percentage of elemental K in each supplement. Available K supplements include K citrate and K gluconate. The amount of elemental K in the supplements is frequently not listed. Instead, they list the weight of the formulation in milligrams per dose. As with Mg, one needs to know the percentage of elemental K+ in each dose listed in milligrams or milliequivalents per dose. Over-the-counter K supplements do not provide significant amounts of elemental K+ per dose. I was on a diuretic and was losing considerable quantities of K through urinary excretion. I needed a prescription from my HCP for an extended-release potassium chloride (KCl). A 10-milliequivalent (meq) or 20-milliequivalent (meq) tablet of extended-release KCl provides 392 milligrams to 782 milligrams of elemental K, respectively (**APPENDIX FOUR**). This equates to one-quarter to one-half of the RDA for elemental K+.

- K supplements alone may not satisfy the RDA for elemental K+. I also consume foods high in elemental K+ content. (**APPENDIX FIVE**).

Abbreviations:
AF= atrial fibrillation
SR= sinus rhythm
Mg= magnesium
K= potassium
Ca- calcium
Na= sodium

CHAPTER ELEVEN: The importance of maintaining hydration to avoid triggering AF.

PLEASE READ THIS CHAPTER BEFORE MOVING ON.

Adequate hydration is frequently advised to maintain good health for many medical conditions. Its relevance as a trigger for AF may be perceived as a repetitive health recommendation, consequently minimizing its importance. A personal experience made me recognize its significance when I recognized dehydration triggered my AF. Before starting this protocol, I experienced AF 39 percent of the time for 7 days. Once it was implemented, my AF eventually converted to SR.

While monitoring my EKGs on a Kardia app, I converted asymptomatically to AF when I contracted bronchitis and a low-grade fever. It made me question the efficacy of my protocol. While convalescing, I read several articles indicating dehydration was a significant trigger of AF. According to a study[5], there is a causal relationship between dehydration and triggering AF in older individuals who had a higher BMI, were on a diuretic, and had a history of heart failure requiring hospitalization. **Almost 10 percent of AF-afflicted individuals are chronically dehydrated, and there is a 2.3 times greater risk for an ischemic stroke in individuals with AF and dehydration compared to AF without dehydration**. Another study[6] compared dehydration in AF-afflicted individuals with comorbid disorders (other significant medical conditions such as diabetes or hypertension) to dehydration in AF-afflicted individuals without comorbid disorders. The AF-afflicted individuals with comorbid disorders had a 60 percent higher risk for ischemic stroke within 10 days following hospital discharge and a 34 percent higher risk for stroke 11-20 days following hospital discharge. This suggests that AF-afflicted individuals who are dehydrated and have comorbid disorders are especially at high risk for a stroke.

I increased my fluids, and within a few days, my AF converted back to SR. My dehydration status was amplified by losing water from my lungs due to bronchitis, the dehydrating effect of fever, and not drinking enough fluids. Dehydration is one of the most important triggers of AF mentioned in **CHAPTER FOUR.** Recognizing that it could increase stroke risk was an inducement for me to maintain hydration.

Dehydration may interfere with efficient functioning of the heart for the following reasons: (1) it can cause a decrease in the size (volume) of heart cells, altering critical concentrations of essential minerals (Mg, K, Na, and Ca) needed for SR; (2) it can alter the three-dimensional structure of enzymes, (i.e., Na/K ATPase), which could affect their functionality, and interfere in energy production required for heart cells, and (3) it can cause an increase in body temperature during vigorous physical activity or from an illness which could result in enzyme denaturation, also interfering in energy production for heart cells.

Detecting dehydration can be difficult unless obvious symptoms are apparent, such as thirst, sweating, fever, or subjective symptoms like dizziness. The most accurate tests for hydration require blood samples, which are expensive and impractical for frequent testing. Although less sensitive, I discovered the best and least costly approach was to purchase dipsticks that detect urine specific gravity. Urine specific gravity (USG) measures the concentration of waste products in urine samples. It reflects how well kidneys dilute or concentrate urine to maintain fluid balance. The specific gravity compares urine to water, which is 1.000. **As a rule, the specific gravity of urine in a well-hydrated individual should be 1.020 or less.**

According to the U.S. National Academies of Sciences, Engineering, and Medicine, adult males should consume about 15 1/2 cups (one cup is equivalent to 8 ounces) of fluids daily, and women approximately 11 1/2 cups daily. Drinking 15 ½ cups daily seemed excessive to me. I reduced the amount to 6 to 7 cups daily if my urine-specific gravity remained 1.020 or less. I monitor my urine-specific gravity once a week.

Abbreviations:
AF= atrial fibrillation
SR= sinus rhythm

CHAPTER TWELVE: The importance of frequent EKG monitoring

<u>EKG monitoring three to four times daily was essential to determine the frequency of my AF, referred to as AF burden</u>. This is defined as the amount of time AF occurs compared to the total time monitored. Using a Holter monitor to obtain EKG data 24/7 is impractical and expensive. Few individuals would consent to wearing them continuously, and they don't provide at-the-moment data to allow immediate changes in this protocol. Without daily monitoring of one's heart rhythm with EKGs, it is difficult to know if conversion to SR is maintained following any intervention, including lifestyle changes. AF can be symptomatic, but the true incidence of AF may be misleading if

asymptomatic AF occurs and is undetected. For this reason, I monitor my EKGs three to four times a day, each for 30 seconds for a total of 2 minutes daily.

The ideal commercial device to monitor EKGs requires the following capabilities:

1. Provide at the moment EKG data

2. Provide AF burden data

3. Provide AF burden data that could be transferred to a computer. This data and occasional lab results measuring Mg and K blood levels helped me determine if changes in supplement formulations or doses were needed.

I identified two monitoring systems/devices for this protocol. Other monitoring devices may be available for this indication, but I had no experience with them.

Apple Watch and iPhone:

1. Provided at-the-moment EKG data.

By clicking on the crown of the Apple Watch, I could view an icon with an EKG electrical symbol for a heartbeat. It opens by tapping on the symbol. It is then necessary to place a finger on the crown and hold it for 30 seconds. At the end of 30 seconds, the watch interprets the EKG, indicating either normal sinus rhythm or AF. The EKG was permanently recorded on the iPhone. I could view it by going to the **HEALTH** icon, **HEART,** and then to **ELECTROCARDIOGRAM (ECG).** Note: ECG is interchangeable with EKG.

2. Provides AF burden data.

It has two methods to calculate AF burden over time frames.

The first is the procedure described in (1), in which EKGs are monitored three to four times daily and recorded on the iPhone. Every week or month, I can open the location for EKGs on the iPhone and count the number of EKGs with AF divided by the total number of EKGs performed in the same time frame.

For the second method, I tapped the **HEALTH** icon on the iPhone, then opened **HEART**, and finally, **AFib History**. I tapped **Set Up**, then **Get Started**, and entered my **Date of Birth**. Next, I selected **Yes** to indicate I was diagnosed with AF by a doctor, and then I tapped **Done**. The graph recorded the percentage of AF at the end of every week. It has the following limitations: (a) it doesn't continuously record the total heart rhythm for a week; (b) I would need to wear the watch 24/7, which is impractical since the watch must be charged nightly; (c) it doesn't provide at-the-moment data; d) if there is no AF is still records a week as <2 percent AF.

3. The EKG data could be transferred to my computer to create a permanent record. I exported each EKG by tapping Export PDF. It was limited if I wanted to export my EKGs for a month as I had to export each EKG separately.

The Kardia app is downloaded on smartphones. Kardia includes a rectangular-shaped metal sensor, which, when touched, will transmit data viewed as EKGs on the iPhone.

1. Provides at-the-moment EKG data

This occurred when I opened the app, tapped on **RECORD YOUR EKG**, and placed my fingers on the Kardia metal sensor shaped like a rectangle that relays the data to the smartphone. The smartphone should be placed on a flat surface above the sensor. There is a V on the metallic sensor. It is important to turn the sensor, so the V is upside down pointing towards the smartphone. The EKG is interpreted and permanently recorded.

2. Provides AF burden data. This required manual calculations.

The app can graph my daily AF history for specified time frames up to thirty-one days. Symbols indicate normal sinus rhythm, sinus rhythm with a wide QRS, bradycardia (slow heart rate), and AF. AF is represented as an orange triangle. When I opened **HEALTH HISTORY**, the app automatically listed a summary of the last 31 days of recorded EKGs and the number of EKGs with AF in the same time frame. I could then calculate the percentage of AF for that current period. If I selected a different 31 days and downloaded the graph, I had to manually count the symbols for AF and divide by the total number of EKGs recorded for that period listed in the top upper corner above the graph.

One problem with Kardia is the orange triangle symbolizing AF has the same color as a different rhythm called *'Sinus rhythm with a wide QRS.'* Individuals with electric conduction defects, such as a complete right bundle branch block, can have a wide QRS. Additionally, several heart medications cans cause a wide QRS, such as but not limited to flecainide and propafenone, lidocaine, and quinidine. The graph cannot differentiate *'Sinus rhythm with a wide QRS'* from *'AF'* since they are viewed as orange triangles.

The AF burden could be determined by viewing the graph for any requested 31 days, counting each recorded EKG with AF in the specified period, and divide by the total number of recorded EKGs.

3. The EKG data was transferred to my computer to create a permanent record.

Neither EKG recording device satisfied all my criteria for an ideal monitoring device. Continuous 24/7 monitoring is currently unavailable on either device, but of the two monitoring devices, the Apple Watch-iPhone almost achieves that on **'Afib HISTORY.'** Its limitations were previously described.

Abbreviations:
AF= atrial fibrillation
SR= sinus rhythm
Mg= magnesium
K= potassium
HRV= % Heart Rate Variability

CHAPTER THIRTEEN: Graph of results (Fig. 2) demonstrating conversion of my AF to SR with My Zebra Treatment Protocol

When I became aware of my AF, a Holter monitor documented I had AF 39 % of the time for 7 days. The common term to define the incidence of AF is AF burden, which refers to the amount of time a person's heart spends in AF compared to the total time monitored. Since most individuals with AF cannot be continuously monitored 24/7, I defined my AF burden (incidence) as the percentage of days per month that I experienced AF. While experimenting with different Mg supplements, my AF burden was detected approximately 20 percent of the days over 6 months. My AF burden decreased to around 3.0 percent of the days during the subsequent 19 months. This occurred while I was on Mg supplements, increased the dose of a K supplement, corrected my dehydration, and ate foods high in Mg and K content. During these 19 months, results from two Holter tests detected no AF for six and seventeen monitored days, respectively.

I included a graph (**Fig. 2**) illustrating my experience with the protocol. **The right Y axis represents the number of days per month I experienced AF which is illustrated by the height of green vertical bars**. The X-axis lists the months from March 2023 to March 2025. My trials with Mg supplements are shown as a horizontal line listing Mg hydroxide, gluconate, and glycinate from April 2023 to March 2024 and Mag-Tab® (Mg L Lactate SR) from April 2024 to March 2025. **The height of** the green vertical bars significantly decreased over the 19 months from September 2023 to March 2025, indicating AF days affected in that period was 3.0 percent compared to the prior six months from March 2023 to August 2023, which was 20.1 percent. Based on an independent statistical analysis, the probability (p) of these results was p= <0.002, meaning the likelihood of this result occurring by chance was extremely low. According to the statistician, this significant result *"provides strong statistical evidence of a decrease in AF incidence"* when comparing the incidence of AF per month for the first 6 month interval (March 2023 to August 2023) to the subsequent 19 month interval (September 2023 to March 2025). **During the first 6 month interval, I experimented with different Mg supplements, and interestingly, there was no consistent reduction in AF until the end of 24** weeks (March 2023 to August 2023). That is compatible with data from a study[25], which indicated oral Mg supplements required 20 to 30 weeks to achieve a steady state of maximum serum Mg concentrations in healthy subjects. It is also consistent with the half-life of Mg[22], which is 6 weeks in humans who are in Mg balance, meaning if they stopped consuming Mg for 6 weeks, it would take 6 weeks to replenish Mg in all cells, including heart cells. However, for AF individuals with pre-existing Mg deficiency in their heart cells, it would likely take multiple Mg half-lives of 6 weeks to achieve replenishment of Mg in all cells, including heart cells.

When comparing the incidence of AF from September 2023 to the end of March 2025, it decreased significantly while I was on several Mg supplements, including Mag-Tab®, from March 2024 to March 2025. I switched to the latter because the manufacturer published data to support its excellent absorption and maintaining stable 24-hour Mg blood levels[18].

During the 19 months from Sept 2023 to the end of March 2025, I experienced three AF recurrences noted by stars and two others not indicated by stars. One was caused by a transient need for more K and was corrected by increasing the K supplement; the second was caused by my reduction in the dose of Mg two times (the 2nd was not shown as a star for one day in July 2024) and both corrected by returning to my previous higher dose of Mg; and the third and most significant was caused by dehydration while experiencing a fever and bronchitis. Another episode of dehydration occurred but is not listed for one day in Jan 2025. All reverted to SR when I hydrated.

The graph also provided data demonstrating a significant statistical relationship between % Heart Rate Variability (% HRV) and the incidence of AF per month. The % HRV was recorded on my iPhone while wearing an Apple Watch without my awareness until I noticed it in August 2024. The % HRV represents the variation in time intervals between heartbeats in milliseconds (msec). **The left Y-axis is the % HRV per month, represented by solid purple vertical bars. The statistician summarized the relationship between the % HRV per month and incidence of AF per month as follows: "** *the median % HRV decreased from 115% to 18.8% (p < 0.001)"* **comparing the % HRV during the first 6 months (March 2023 to August 2023) to the subsequent 19 months**

(September 2023 to March 2025), respectively. To further emphasize, the statistician stated: *"Overall, AF incidence and % HRV have a strong positive correlation of r=0.750 with a p< 0.001."* Hence, when the % HRV was low (minimal variation or attenuated), there was a strong correlation with a low incidence of AF. Additionally, when the % HRV became unattenuated, it would signal AF recurrence. **CHAPTER NINE** provides scientific literature that supports this conclusion. **Fig.1** are graphs demonstrating unattenuated and attenuated % HRV.

During the incubation period in AF (March' 23 to August '23), my EKGs exhibited other electrical conduction defects, called left anterior fascicular block and second-degree Mobitz type-1. They indicated defective electrical conduction that might require a pacemaker. Fortunately, both disappeared while on my protocol.

I am aware of the limitations regarding my data and conclusions. First, the most obvious is reporting data that only included one person. As I mentioned, being a physician with a scientific background, I have been as objective as possible reporting the data, some of which was recorded independently on my iPhone/Apple Watch without my awareness (% HRV), and the incidence of AF weekly from August 2024 to the end of March 2025. During the 25 months of self-observation, I tried to control lifestyle factors that might exacerbate AF. I experienced no weight change or BMI reduction during that period and did my best to reduce stress. There were no new medical conditions or changes to existing ones. Also, there were no new medications or dose changes of existing ones that could have affected these results, **CHAPTER NINE**.

During the 25 months, I changed the type and dose of Mg supplements, increased the K dose, and addressed dehydration. One could argue not keeping these variables constant could affect the outcome. My response to those reasonable concerns is AF reappeared several times, indicating it never disappeared. Mainly, it demonstrates that my protocol controlled my AF but did not cure it.

It is difficult to compare the recurrence rate of my asymptomatic, long-standing persistent AF treated with my protocol to the recurrence rates of common interventions for symptomatic and asymptomatic AF-afflicted individuals. All current interventions have significant recurrence rates (**APPENDIX ONE**). Most interventions do not include follow-up with daily EKGs to detect asymptomatic AF. The difference between conventional interventions and my protocol is the latter has a lower risk and cost and more accurately recognizes asymptomatic AF recurrences with daily EKG monitoring.

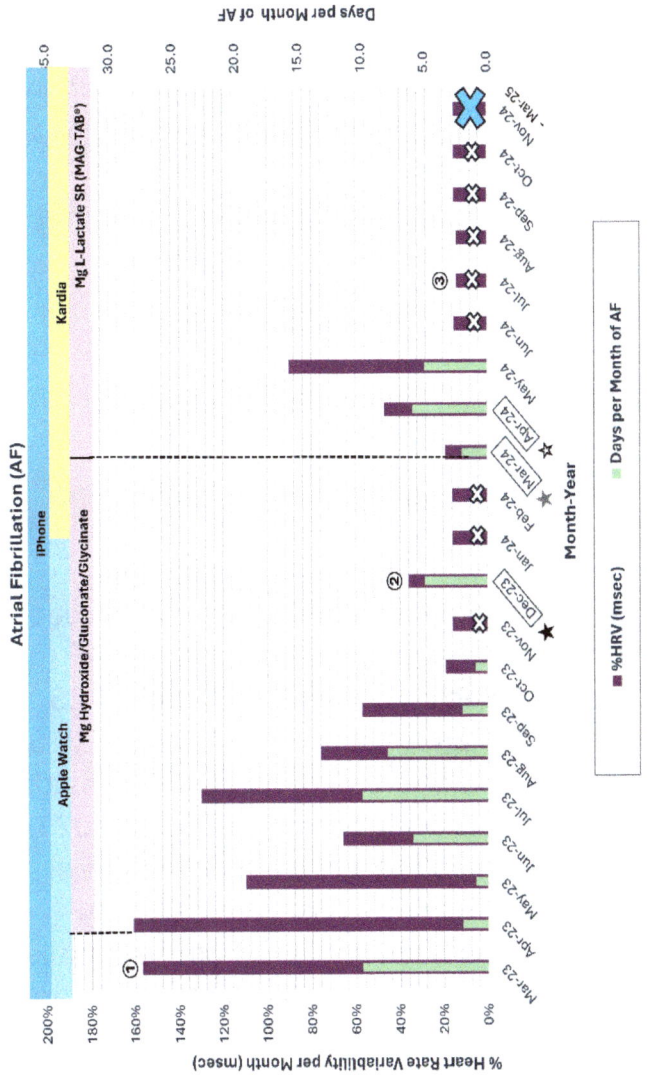

Fig. 2 Chart illustrating incidence of AF and correlation with % HRV

Legend	
★ Dec-23	Increased KCL
★ Mar-24	Corrected by readjusting Mag-Tab dose
☆ Apr-24	Respiratory infection /corrected dehydration
✖	AF undetected
✖ (large)	AF undetected (multiple months)

Holter Monitor Results	
①	7 days detected 39% of the time
②	undetected for 7 days
③	undetected for 13 days

Fig. 2: Graph demonstrating significant reduction in the incidence of AF days per month of AF (green bars) from September 2023 to March 2025 compared to prior six months of March 2023 to August 2023, (p=<.002). The graph indicates that from March 2023 to the end of August 2023, an incubation period of approximately 24 weeks on oral Mg supplements was observed before AF consistently converted to SR from September 2023 to March 2025. This is consistent with an article[25] indicating even for healthy subjects, the incubation required to achieve a steady state of maximum serum Mg concentrations is between 20 to 30 weeks. It supports several half-lives of Mg (6 weeks each) are likely required to replenish Mg deficiency

in AF individuals with preexisting Mg deficiency in their heart cells.

The graph demonstrates a direct correlation between the % HRV per month (purple bars) and days per month of AF (green bars). Statistician's analysis is " *the median % HRV decreased from 115% to 18.8% (p < 0.001)*" comparing the % HRV during the first six months (March 2023 to August 2023) to the subsequent 19 months (September 2023 to March 2025), respectively. *"Overall, AF incidence and percent change of HRV have a strong positive correlation of r=0.750 with a p< 0.001."* It suggests that if the % HRV suddenly increased from its baseline, there is a likelihood my AF recurred. The high % HRV in May 2024 represents an overlap from the 1 week recurrence of AF in late April to two weeks in May 2024. **Fig.1** illustrates unattenuated and attenuated % HRV.

Abbreviations
AF= atrial fibrillation
Mg = magnesium
K = potassium
SR= sinus rhythm
AFL= atrial flutter
HCP = healthcare professional
RDA= recommended daily allowance

CHAPTER FOURTEEN: Outline of My Zebra Treatment Protocol and its associated risks.

The following outlines the low-risk, low-cost protocol that has converted my AF to SR with long-term oral Mg supplements, K supplements, and hydration. A part of this protocol emphasizes that I remained in contact with my HCPs, who are familiar with my medical conditions and medications.

Clinical criteria for implementation of My Zebra Treatment Protocol.

- This protocol was effective for my asymptomatic, long-standing, persistent AF. Retrospectively, I could not predict my protocol would have been effective if I:

- had experienced symptomatic AF;
- had paroxysmal AF, meaning my symptoms lasted up to 7 days;
- had been classified as having permanent AF;
- had been previously treated with any of the conventional interventions described in **Chapter TWO,** to convert my AF to SR. I would not have known if the protocol could prevent recurrences of AF and maintain SR;
- needed elective heart surgery, and whether it would have prevented postoperative AF if administered at least 20 to 30 weeks before the surgery;
- had experienced atrial flutter (AFL) and whether it would have converted to SR based on observations in article[12] cited in **CHAPTER SIX.**

- My protocol was compatible with my medical conditions and concurrent medications. I did not have: chronic kidney disease, although I remain aware that AF can cause this condition; co-existing cardiovascular diseases such as coronary artery disease, cardiac valve disorders, and hypertension; hyperthyroidism (increased thyroid activity); a history of bradycardia (low heart rate defined as less than 60 beats per minute) and/or hypotension(less than 90/60) because Mg could exacerbate both and lead to dizziness and fainting; I was aware of drug interactions with Mg mentioned in **CHAPTER FOUR.**

- I addressed predisposing factors that could increase my incidence of AF[3,49], **CHAPTER FOUR**

- I was aware of potential risks associated with

this protocol (listed below).

Outline of My Zebra Treatment Protocol:

I sought advice from my HCP while implementing this protocol.

- **Anticoagulant.** <u>My HCP advised me to remain on an anticoagulant. Deciding to stop the anticoagulant would require a decision by my HCP.</u>

- **Monitoring my EKGs three to four times daily.** **CHAPTER TWELVE** explains the pros and cons of different EKG monitoring devices. I also followed my % Heart Rate Variability (% HRV) as a parameter that appeared to correlate with the incidence of my AF and, consequently, a potential marker for AF recurrences, **CHAPTER NINE**.

- **Baseline tests**: I requested the following baseline tests from my HCPs. Mg and other electrolyte blood levels (K, Na, Ca), serum creatinine (to monitor hydration and if chronic kidney disease occurred as a complication of AF). An EKG was done before I started oral Mg supplements to determine my baseline QTc. All blood tests were repeated within a month or two after starting my protocol, ideally every four months for the first year and every six months. A repeat EKG was requested 6 months after starting the Mg supplement and annually to determine if there was reduction in the QTc interval.

- **Special imaging tests to determine if blood clots existed in my heart.** My HCP requested a transthoracic echocardiogram (TTE) and a CTA angiogram. The latter was primarily to make sure my coronary blood vessels were unobstructed. Another test that would more definitively rule out a blood clot in my heart is called a transesophageal echocardiogram (TEE).

Measured urine-specific gravity once a week to determine if it is 1.020 or less to confirm adequate hydration.

- **Lifestyle optimization** to minimize or eliminate predisposing factors for my AF[3,49]. **CHAPTER FOUR.**

- **Consumed foods high in Mg and K content.** I was aware my Mg and K supplements could not fulfill my RDA . Consequently, I consumed foods fortified in both. (**APPENDICES THREE AND FIVE**).

- **Selection of Mg supplements**
  - One Mg supplement[18] has been used in several peer-reviewed clinical studies[17,24,41,42]. It has excellent absorption of 40 percent; is slow-release; achieves rapid onset of action in 3 hours with stabilized therapeutic blood levels by 3 days maintained over twenty-four-hour

intervals[17]; can normalize Mg deficiency in hearts of AF-afflicted individuals [16,17]; has minimal gastrointestinal discomfort; and is manufactured with quality control. The manufacturer has published pharmacokinetic data to support these claims[18]. This slow-release product is Mg L-Lactate (Mag-Tab®; Niche Pharmaceuticals, LLC, see **DISCLOSURE at the beginning of the book.** One caplet of Mag-Tab provides 84 mg of elemental Mg. I started with one-half caplet morning and evening and monitored my heart rhythm by viewing EKGs on my Apple Watch-iPhone or Kardia app three to four times daily. If the EKG remained in AF, I increased the dose by one-half caplet in the AM or PM up to 1 caplet twice daily. There is no recommended maximum dose for this preparation. As a precaution, I would obtain a repeat Mg serum level before I increased above one caplet twice daily. My daily dose was one and one-half caplets in the morning and one in the evening. I reduced the dose if gastrointestinal side effects became problematic. One clinical study with this product administered three caplets every twelve hours for three doses with minimal side effects except for occasional gastrointestinal discomfort.[17] The authors observed that *"the quick onset…with Mg L Lactate, acute use of the oral product…may be possible and would obviate the need for intravenous access."* **The author is referring to Mag-Tab® by Niche Pharmaceuticals. If validated, this formulation could reduce the incubation time needed to replenish Mg in heart cells.**

- In earlier months, while developing this protocol, I administered other organic supplements that contained only one Mg supplement without other ingredients. Some were manufactured with quality control cGMP, and ideally had data proving good absorption. I experimented with Mg gluconate and glycinate, as seen in the graph (**Fig. 2**) in **CHAPTER THIRTEEN**. The incidence of my AF significantly reduced after 24 weeks on oral Mg supplements. I discontinued them to try Mag-Tab because of published scientific data supporting its use. Other organic Mg supplements with decent absorption might be effective, but I did not try them. Mg aspartate has 40 percent absorption[28]. Other Mg supplements that might be effective are Mg malate, and Mg citrate. One inorganic Mg supplement I did not try with good absorption is Mg Chloride.

- **K supplementation**. I was on a diuretic. My HCP prescribed an extended-release formulation of K chloride tablets (20 meq), which provides one-half (780 mg) of the total RDA for elemental K which is 1560 mg. I was aware AF is associated with K deficiency[9], so I added it and made sure I ate foods fortified in K content.

- **Monitoring my heart rhythm with my Apple Watch-iPhone or Kardia app**. This is an essential feature of my protocol. Even if I had symptomatic AF, I might not know I had intervals of asymptomatic AF unless I monitored my heart rhythm daily. I have been asymptomatic, and without monitoring my daily EKGs, I would not know when to make changes in my protocol. I maintained Mg/K doses if SR occurred.

However, if SR reverted to AF, I increased the dose of the Mg supplement slowly, preferably with Mag-Tab, because it is rapidly absorbed and maintains stable concentrations over 24-hour intervals. Repeated Mg/K blood levels were obtained if Mg/K doses were changed. I also maintained adequate hydration. The maximum dose of Mag-Tab is not stated, but one study had subjects on three caplets twice daily for three days without significant side effects[17]. Another study[42] treated patients with Mag-Tab (three caplets twice daily for 12 months). Approximately 28% of the patients dropped out because of the large number of pills and diarrhea side effects.

- **Titrating the dose of Mg and K was based on EKG interpretations, Mg and K blood levels, symptoms due to potential Mg/K toxicity, symptoms related to AF, and discomfort**

caused by Mg-induced gastrointestinal side effects. I remained in contact with my HCPs regarding any concerns.

- **Incubation time administering oral Mg supplements**: I required 24 weeks to convert my AF to SR. This was compatible with literature described in **CHAPTER SEVEN**, noting the half-life of Mg is 6 weeks for someone in Mg balance, but it would likely require multiple 6-week half-lives of Mg to replenish pre-existing Mg deficiency in heart cells of individuals with AF. Data indicates it may take between 20 to 30 weeks[25] to maintain maximum blood levels of Mg, even in healthy individuals. Based on observations in a clinical study[17] in which the onset of action for Mag-Tab (Mg-Lactate SR) was 3 hours up to 3 days, if I had administered this formulation earlier, it may have reduced the time required to convert my AF to SR.`

- **Potential risks implementing My Zebra Treatment Protocol:**
  - This is an elective protocol, and I would not have implemented it if I had experienced severe AF symptoms requiring immediate intervention with other treatments.
  - During its implementation, because of the extended incubation time needed to determine its efficacy, I could have experienced a spontaneous stroke unrelated to the implementation of my protocol.
  - The risk for a stroke If my AF converted to SR still existed when compared with someone who has always been in SR[4]. However, converting from AF to SR reduced my stroke risk compared to remaining in AF[4].

- Remaining in SR one hundred percent of the time did not occur with this protocol. I realized my stroke risk could increase when and if I had a recurrence of AF.
- Toxicity from elevated Mg and/or K blood levels is rare but could occur. For that reason, I had periodic Mg and K blood levels. I maintained awareness of symptoms caused by elevated Mg, which include low blood pressure and/or slow heart rate, dizziness or fainting, fatigue, nausea, vomiting, and muscle weakness. Symptoms of elevated K are muscle fatigue, nausea, weakness, and abnormal heart rhythms that can be life-threatening.
- The following is a potential complication that occurs rarely with all AF interventions, including anti-arrhythmic medications,

electrical cardioversion, and catheter ablation procedures. I was aware it could potentially occur with this treatment protocol. Conversion of AF to SR could dislodge a clot residing in my heart and cause a stroke. Countering this unlikely occurrence with this protocol is by not trying to convert my AF to SR, I had a higher risk for a stroke, even on an anti-coagulant.

Abbreviations
AF= atrial fibrillation
Mg= magnesium
K = potassium
SR= sinus rhythm
HCP = healthcare professional
RDA- recommended daily allowance

CHAPTER FIFTEEN: Key points I learned from implementing My Zebra Treatment Protocol.

- **There is compelling scientific evidence indicating Mg and K deficiencies correlate with increased incidence of AF;**

- **Blood testing to determine Mg deficiency is not always predictable;**
    - **A normal blood (serum) Mg blood level does not rule out Mg deficiency since the blood circulation represents only one percent of the total Mg stores in the body;**
    - **A low serum Mg may indicate significant Mg deficiency;**

- There is evidence of low Mg concentrations inside heart cells of AF-afflicted individuals even with a normal Mg blood level.

- There are observations K deficiency may be accompanied by Mg deficiency, and to correct this, it may be necessary to increase Mg supplementation;

- **CHAPTER FOURTEEN** indicates my asymptomatic long-standing persistent AF, and medical history/medications were compatible with being a candidate for my protocol. However, **CHAPTER FOURTEEN** outlines criteria that might have excluded my candidacy for this protocol.

- I remain aware of the potential side effects associated with my protocol, outlined in CHAPTER FOURTEEN.

- Before implementing my protocol, I involved my HCP and requested the following screening tests: Mg and K blood levels, creatinine blood levels for hydration and kidney status, and an EKG to measure the QTc interval. My HCP made sure I had no existing blood clots in my heart by ordering imaging tests discussed in CHAPTER FOURTEEN.

- When I first became aware of AF, my HCP started me on an anticoagulant. The HCP recommended I remain on it even though I was in SR because a recurrence of AF would increase my stroke risk.

- I was aware not to delay alternative AF treatments if I had an emergency need for their implementation.

- I made sure I eliminated predisposing factors (CHAPTER FOUR) that might increase my incidence of AF;

- Data indicates replenishment of Mg with oral supplements requires an extended time between <u>6 weeks or up to 20 to 30 weeks</u>.

- There are two approaches to replenish my Mg deficiency. First, I consume the recommended dietary allowance (RDA) in foods high in Mg content. <u>Second is selection of a Mg supplement with excellent absorption, rapid onset of action, maintains therapeutic blood levels over 24-hour intervals, and is manufactured by cGMP</u>

standards (CHAPTERS EIGHT & FOURTEEN; APPENDIX FOUR). Currently, one product fulfills these criteria with published documentation, namely slow-release Mg L-Lactate (Mag-Tab®; Niche Pharmaceuticals, LLC[18].

- My K deficiency is addressed with K supplements and foods high in K content, especially while on a diuretic.

- I remain vigilant about hydration because I would be at a greater risk of ischemic stroke if I became dehydrated. I monitor my urine-specific gravity once a week. My threshold for remaining hydrated is a urine-specific gravity of 1.020 or less.

- I keep a record of EKGs and the Mg/K supplements .

- I keep a permanent record every 30 days and dose and type of Mg/K supplements. I would record any new medications, especially heart and blood pressure-related medications.

- I monitor my EKGs three to four times a day and, if possible, after exercise. Repeat monitoring can reveal when my EKG converts to SR or if AF recurs.

- I remained on the same Mg supplement for at least six weeks. If I remained in AF or converted from SR to AF, I would consider the following options:

    ❖ Add incremental doses of the same Mg supplement to increase the amount of elemental Mg and repeat my Mg blood level a few weeks later.

- ❖ Add a long-acting K supplement if I have no evidence of chronic kidney disease.

- ❖ Consider continuing my protocol for 20 to 30 weeks.

- ❖ If I didn't convert to SR, I would consider selecting a different Mg supplement and repeat the first step.

- ❖ My protocol emphasizes that I titrate the dose of Mg and K based on EKG interpretations, Mg and K blood levels, symptoms related to AF, symptoms caused by potential Mg/K toxicity, and Mg gastrointestinal side effects. I would contact my HCP if I needed expertise related to these issues.

- Initially, as mentioned, I requested a Mg blood level before starting my treatment protocol and repeated it approximately every 4-6 months to ensure it was normal. I remained aware of symptoms suggesting Mg toxicity.

- I also obtained a blood K level when starting the K supplement and repeated it approximately every 4-6 months. I remained aware of symptoms suggesting K toxicity.

- Although I do not have chronic kidney disease, I am aware I could develop it as a complication of AF. I monitor my kidney function by requesting an annual or bi-annual blood creatinine test and checking my blood K levels to avoid K toxicity.

- **Finally, I remained involved with my HCPs whenever significant issues or changes in my protocol were needed.**

CHAPTER SIXTEEN: A unified theory explaining why inflammation and Mg deficiency cause AF; the involvement of an uncontrolled immune mechanism causing the inflammation; how unhealthy lifestyles stimulate this immune mechanism; and why replenishing Mg may reverse AF to SR

Abbreviations
AF= atrial fibrillation
SR= sinus rhythm
Na= sodium
K= potassium
Mg=magnesium
Ca= calcium

There is considerable interest in chronic inflammation as an underlying cause of AF. The theory is based on two levels of evidence.

First, there are changes in the structure of the heart of an individual affected by AF, referred to as anatomical remodeling. Biopsies of heart tissue obtained from AF-afflicted individuals reveal fibrosis (scarring) and changes associated with inflammation, such as calcifications, thickening of atrial walls, and disarray of organized heart cell arrangement. The changes can alter normal electrical conduction pathways and promote AF. The anatomical changes can progress over time and partly explain why individuals with persistent (up to one year) and long-standing persistent AF (more than one year) become less responsive to therapeutic interventions.

The second line of evidence involves elevated blood markers of inflammation. One particular marker is high-sensitivity C-reactive protein (hs-CRP). It is a very sensitive marker of inflammation and can be increased in an assortment of acute and chronic inflammatory conditions, such as infectious diseases, heart attacks, obesity, autoimmune conditions (lupus and rheumatoid arthritis), cancers, and reactions to medications. My assessment is this blood test may only be a reliable marker for inflammation in AF-afflicted individuals when other causes for its elevation are excluded.

To date, no unified theory exists to explain the cause of inflammation underlying AF. One of the most interesting theories is based on the involvement of a relatively new mechanism of innate (born with) immunity, the NLRP-3 inflammasome mentioned in the **INTRODUCTION**.[43-45] The protein (cryopyrin) comprising the NLRP-3 is located inside specialized immune cells and heart cells (cardiomyocytes[43]). Evolutionarily, its presence provides humans with survival capacity to stave off pathogens on first exposure. Its other function is to protect organs from damage caused by dying cells due to aging processes and ischemic insults (loss of blood supply as in a heart attack). It differs from acquired immunity, which humans develop after first exposure to pathogens or from vaccinations.

The NLRP-3 inflammasome is stimulated by danger signals, such as molecules spilling out of dying cells (ATP, proteins, metabolites) and molecules that crystallize derived from metabolism (cholesterol, saturated fatty acids, and uric acid). When stimulated, the NLRP-3 secretes cytokines (small proteins) that attract inflammatory cells, resulting in acute and chronic inflammation. Unhealthy lifestyles that predispose to AF (excessive alcohol, obesity, diabetes mellitus type 2, smoking) can stimulate the NLRP-3. Obesity and diabetes Type 2 are associated with increased levels of saturated fatty acids, cholesterol, and uric acids, which crystallize and can stimulate the NLRP-3. Nicotine can stimulate NLRP-3 in cells lining the bronchial tree. Alcohol stimulates the NLRP-3 by its metabolites. Some triggers of the NLRP-3 are listed in red in **CHAPTER FOUR**, which can be controlled by lifestyle changes and appropriate medications that lower cholesterol, fatty acids, and uric acid. Recommendations that unhealthy lifestyles can cause AF may not be enough to motivate individuals with AF. However, they may become more motivated by understanding unhealthy lifestyles may fuel an immune mechanism that could cause the inflammation underlying AF.

The inflammation resulting from the secretion of cytokines by the NLRP-3 can be unchecked, resulting in chronic inflammation and damage to the heart, especially pacemaker cells, leading to AF. Currently, research efforts are in progress to inhibit NLRP-3 and reduce the inflammatory response that can damage the heart. An article previously mentioned in the **INTRODUCTION** demonstrated that inhibiting NLRP-3 could prevent AF in mice genetically predisposed to AF[2]. An extensive review of this subject[43] supports the notion that activation of the NLRP-3 can cause inflammation in heart cells, especially the upper chambers of the heart (atria), and cause AF. Assuming NLRP-3 inhibitor medications are proven safe and efficacious for individuals with AF, they may eventually lead to an effective treatment and potentially a cure for AF.

One of the most biologically active cytokines secreted by the NLRP-3 is interleukin-1β (IL-1β). Evidence indicates IL-1β can inhibit critical enzymes (Na^+/K^+ ATPase)[44] in heart cells required for energy production. These enzymes break down a molecule called ATP that stores energy. Inhibition of these energy-generating enzymes may cause pacemaker cells to not function because energy is required to maintain electrolyte pumps (**CHAPTER FIVE**) needed to generate SR electrical impulses. Another reason there may be an energy deficit in pacemaker cells is that Mg must combine with and change the chemical structure of ATP so ATPase enzymes can break it down for energy production. Consequently, the combination of IL-1β inhibition of ATPase enzymes and a deficiency of Mg in heart cells of AF individuals could create an energy deficit that prevents SR electrical impulse generation from pacemaker cells. This allows aberrant cells in the left atrium to takeover to develop AF.

One might ask if there is a biological advantage for IL-1β inhibition of energy-producing enzymes in heart cells. My best guess is IL-1β, by inhibiting energy production in aging cells, may enhance their programmed death and removal as part of the regenerative process. However, if there is significant cell damage and death, excessive IL-1β production may occur and cause chronic inflammation and inhibition of critical ATPase enzymes. Reversing this inhibition may occur by increasing Mg concentrations inside heart cells, which allows Mg to combine and change the structure of ATP in order for ATPase to break it down for energy production. Consequently, Mg replenishment in heart cells could optimize energy production, restore electrolyte pumps, and reactivate pacemaker cells to produce SR. Adding K supplementation is understandable when recognizing K is lost from intracellular compartments due to the death of heart cells from aging or ischemia.

In summary, inhibiting the NLRP-3 inflammasome and replenishing Mg in the heart cells could control or potentially cure AF. Hopefully, my theory will stimulate dialogues within medical academia.

CHAPTER SEVENTEEN: Final comments.

As a physician and scientist, I have tried to objectively record my observations in my auto-cardiography. What I experienced could be an occurrence that will only benefit me and may be perceived as an anecdotal observation; however, the rationale for my protocol is based on evidence in scientific articles cited in this book. Moreover, evaluation of my data by an independent Ph.D. statistician provided evidential corroboration for my protocol. American and European cardiology guidelines[3,49] for AF do not mention oral Mg supplementation as a potential intervention for converting AF to SR. Recently, a review article[46] on AF also did not mention oral Mg supplementation as an option for treating AF. Despite its absence, it is my hope this book will encourage random control trials to determine if my protocol could be an effective therapy for individuals with asymptomatic persistent or long-standing persistent AF.

The collaborative research between Dr. Hal Hoffman and me[47] led to the discovery of the cryopyrin protein, which other researchers subsequently recognized as the essential protein in the NLRP-3 inflammasome. Medications capable of inhibiting the NLRP-3 in individuals with AF may provide the foundation for effective therapy for AF. **(CHAPTER SIXTEEN).**

Recognizing a Mg-containing laxative that might correlate with my EKG conversion to SR was an epiphany. It led to the 'outside the box' Zebra Treatment Protocol supported by underappreciated scientific observations. I conclude with a quote from 'His Last Bow: An Epilogue of Sherlock Holmes'. *"It has been an axiom of mine that the little things are infinitely the most important."* Perhaps the *"little things"* in my protocol made the difference in successfully treating my AF.

APPENDIX ONE: Medical consequences associated with AF interventions.

Cardioversion risks with antiarrhythmic medications:

- New or worsening arrhythmias. One is life-threatening, called torsade de pointes
- Dislodged blood clot causing a stroke
- Slow heart rate
- Low blood pressure
- May not be effective
- Other complications depend on the medication being used (see internet).

*The estimated recurrence rate varies between forty to seventy percent depending on the medication.

Electric Cardioversion risks:
- Dislodged blood clots can cause stroke
- Other less dangerous heart rhythms
- Skin burns
- Temporary low blood pressure
- Heart failure

*The estimated recurrence rate varies between sixty-three to eighty-four percent.

Cardiac ablation risks[3]:

- Bleeding or infection at the site where the catheter was inserted;
- Blood vessel damage and bleeding. Occurs in 1.4% of patients;

- Coronary artery spasms leading to heart attacks;
- Kidney failure due to shredding of red blood cells;
- Heart valve damage;
- Fistula (passage) between the esophagus and left atrium. Estimated to occur between 0.015 % and 0.25 % of patients;
- Pericardial tamponade (blood in the sac surrounding the heart), occurs between 0.8%[45] and 2% of patients;
- New or worsening arrhythmia;
- Slow heart rate that could require a pacemaker to correct;
- Nerve paralysis (phrenic and vagal nerves. Estimated phrenic nerve paralysis occurs from 5-10% for cryoballoon ablation;
- Blood clots that can dislodge, causing a stroke
- Narrowing of the veins that carry blood between the lungs and heart (pulmonary vein stenosis);
- Damage to the kidneys from contrast used during the procedure;
- Potential of micro-bubbles in the left atrium that could potentially cause brain lesions (associated with PFA);
- Rare deaths related to the procedure is 0.06% or 6 out of 10,000 procedures;
- Death risk if general anesthesia is required is 1 out of 100,000 surgical procedures;
- Outcomes are worse for individuals 75 or older

*The estimated recurrence rate varies between twenty to fifty percent depending on the procedure and if recurrence occurs early within three months, late within one year, or very late after one year.

*There is literature[48] suggesting a newer ablation procedure, pulsed-field ablation, may have fewer complications, specifically less injury to the esophagus and phrenic nerve (damage to the phrenic nerve can lead to diaphragm paralysis, making it difficult to breathe);
** Studies suggest ablation, in general, may lower the risk for stroke in some patients with asymptomatic AF, particularly those with a high risk for stroke, based on factors of age, hypertension, diabetes, and other heart conditions.

Maze surgery risks:
- Bleeding;
- Blood clots;
- Infection;
- Complications from anesthesia;
- Arrhythmias;
- Kidney failure;
- Other organ failure;
- Death related to the procedure itself;
- Death related to general anesthesia is 1 out of 100,000;

* The recurrence rate of AF varies depending on studies. One study described AF recurrence of 14.2% at seven years and 26.5% when patients were not taking antiarrhythmic drugs. Another study found that 35.4% of patients had a recurrence after six months, and 74.9% had a recurrence after seven years.

Walkman procedure
- Strokes from the device by causing clotting;

- Almost the same risks listed for catheter ablation;
- Death risk for general anesthesia is 1 out of 100,000 surgical procedures;

APPENDIX TWO: Recommended Daily Allowance (RDA) for milligrams (mgs) of elemental Mg per day. Resource from the National Institute of Health.

Children

1-3 years	80 mg
4-8 years	130 mg
9-13 years	240 mg
Teen boys 14-18 years	410 mg
Teen girls 14-18 years	360 mg
Men	420 mg
Women	320 mg
Pregnant women	350 mg

APPENDIX THREE: Foods with high Mg content

Resource
https://www.nal.usda.gov/sites/www.nal.usda.gov/files/magnesium.pdf

Foods Containing Mg	Serving Size	Elemental Mg in milligrams
Pumpkin seeds, hulled, roasted	1 ounce	150
Halibut, cooked	3 ounces	90
Almonds, dry roasted	1 ounce	80
Cashews, dry roasted	1 ounce	75
Soybeans, mature, cooked	½ cup	75
***Spinach, frozen, cooked**	½ cup	75
Nuts, mixed, dry roasted	1 ounce	65
Cereal, shredded wheat	2 rectangular biscuits	55
Oatmeal, instant, fortified, prepared with water	1 cup	55
Potato, baked with skin	1 medium	50
Peanuts, dry roasted	1 ounce	50
Peanut butter, smooth	2 tablespoons	50
Wheat bran, crude	2 tablespoons	45
Black-eyed peas, cooked	½ cup	45

Foods Containing Mg	**Serving Size**	**Elemental Mg in milligrams**
Yogurt, plain, skim milk	8 fluid ounces	45
Bran flakes	½ cup	40
Vegetarian baked beans	½ cup	40
Rice, brown, long grained, cooked	½ cup	40
Lentils, mature seeds, cooked	½ cup	35
Avocado, California	½ cup pureed	35
Kidney beans, canned	½ cup	35
Pinto beans, cooked	½ cup	35
Wheat germ, crude	2 tablespoons	35
Chocolate milk	1 cup	33
Banana, raw	1 medium	30
Milk chocolate candy bar	1.5-ounce bar	28
Milk, reduced fat (2%) or fat-free	1 cup	27
Bread, whole wheat, commercially prepared	1 slice	25

***Now you know why *Popeye the Sailor* ate spinach**

APPENDIX FOUR: Chart for Mg and K Supplements

LONG-ACTING SLOW RELEASE ORGANIC Mg SALT	% of elemental Mg in each supplement	Weight of one dose of each Mg formulation listed in milligrams (mg)	mgs of elemental Mg in one dose of a supplement
Mg L-Lactate Mag-Tab® SR ; Niche Pharmaceuticals	10	contains 840 mg of Mg L Lactate	84 mg
SHORT-ACTING Mg SALTS (organic and non-organic)			
ORGANIC Mg SALTS			
Mg aspartate	8	100 to 500 mg	8 to 40 mg
Mg lactate	8-10	100 to 500 mg	8 to 40 mg
Mg citrate	5	100 to 500 Mg	5 to 25 mg
Mg gluconate	7	500 to 1000 mg	35 to 70 mg
Mg glycinate	12	100 to 500 mg	12 to 60 mg
Mg malate	10	400 to 1000 mg	40 to 100 mg
Mg picolinate	9	50 to 200 mg	5 to 18 mg
Mg pidolate	10	402 to 500 mg	40 to 50 mg
Mg taurate	10	125 to 1500 mg	12.5 to 150 mg
Mg L-threonate	12	500 to 2000 mg	60 to 240 mg
INORGANIC Mg SALTS			
Mg oxide	60	140 to 500 mg	84 to 300 mg
Mg hydroxide (contained in Milk of Magnesia, a laxative)	41	400 to 1200 mg	134 to 492 mg
Mg chloride	25	535 mg	134 mg
Mg carbonate	29	250 mg	73 mg

POTASSIUM (K)	% of elemental K in each dose	Weight of one dose	Elemental K in one dose
Potassium gluconate	18	550 mg	99 mg
Potassium Citrate	13	200 mg	26 mg
Potassium Chloride ER (extended-release)	52 for (20 meq) 52 for (10 meq)	1491 mg 746 mg	775 mg 372 mg

LEGEND

Supplements I am currently administering

Supplements with good absorption based on reports in medical literature

Supplements I administered until switching to Mag-Tab ® SR illustrated in **Fig.2**

APPENDIX FIVE: Foods with high K content

Fruits: Bananas, melons, oranges, nectarines, kiwi, mango, papaya, prunes, pomegranate, dates, dried fruits, dried figs

Vegetables:

Avocados, broccoli, brussels sprouts, sweet potatoes, parsnips, pumpkin, vegetable juices, white potatoes, winter squash

Tomato and tomato-based products

Deep-colored and leafy green vegetables (such as spinach or Swiss chard)

Dried beans and peas, black beans, refried beans, baked beans, lentils, legumes

Other

Milk, yogurt • Nuts and seeds • Bran and bran products • Chocolate, granola, molasses, peanut butter

Bibliography

1. Hoffman HM, Mueller JL, Brodie DH, Wanderer AA, Kolodner RD: Mutation of a new gene encoding a putative pyrin-like protein causes cold autoinflammatory syndrome and Muckle-Wells syndrome. Nature Genetics. 2001, 29: 301-5.

2. Yao C, Veleva T, Scott L Jr et al. Enhanced Cardiomyocyte NLRP3 Inflammasome Signaling Promotes Atrial Fibrillation. Circulation. 2018 Nov 13;138(20):2227-2242.

3. Joglar JA, Chung MK, Ambruster AL et al. 2023 ACC/AHA/ACCP/HRS Guideline for the Diagnosis and Management of AF: A Report of the American College of Cardiology/ American Heart Association Joint Committee on Clinical Practice Guidelines. Circulation. 2024;149: e 1-e156.

4. Adderley N, Niranthakumar K, Marshal T. Risk of stroke and transient ischaemic attack in patients with a diagnosis of resolved AF: retrospective cohort studies. BMJ 2018; 360:k1717.

5. Chuda A, Kaszkowiak M, Banach M, et.al. The relationship of dehydration and body mass index with the occurrence of AF in heart failure patients. Front Cardiovasc Med. 2021, 8: 668653.

6. Swerdel J, Janevic T, Kostis W, et al. Association between dehydration and short-

term risk of ischemic stroke in patients with AF. Transl Stroke Res. 2017;8:122-130.

7. Li J, Agarwal S, Alonso A. . Airflow Obstruction, Lung Function, and Incidence of AF. The Atherosclerosis Risk in Communities (ARIC) Study. Circulation. 2014;129:971-980.

8. Biesenbach P, Martensson J, Lucchetta L, ,et.al. Pharmacokinetics of magnesium bolus therapy in cardiothoracic surgery. J Cardiothorac Vase Anesth 2018, 32:11289-1294.

9. Krijthe BP, Heeringa J, Kors JA, et al. Serum potassium levels and the risk of AF: the Rotterdam Study. Int J Cardiol. 2013;168(6):5411-5415. doi:10.1016/j.ijcard.2013.08.04.

10. Whang R, Flink EB, DycknerT. Magnesium Depletion as a Cause of Refractory Potassium Repletion. Arch Intern Med.1985, 145: 1686-1689.

11. Khan AM, Lubitz SA, Sullivan LM.et.al. Low serum magnesium and the development of AF in the community: the Framingham Heart Study. Circulation 2013 Jan 1;127(1):33-8.

12. Nielsen FH, Milne DB, Klevay LM, et.al. Dietary magnesium deficiency induces heart rhythm changes, impairs glucose tolerance, and decreases serum cholesterol in postmenopausal women. J Am Coll Nutr. 2007; 26:121–132.

13. Markovits, N, Kurnik, D., Halkin, H, et. Al. Database evaluation of the association between serum magnesium levels and the risk of AF in the community. Int. J. Cardiol. 2016, 205, 142–146.

14. Misialek JR, Lopez FL, Lutsey P, et.al. Serum and dietary magnesium and incidence of AF in whites and in African Americans-- Atherosclerosis Risk in Communities (ARIC) study. Circ J, 2013;77(2):323-9.

15. Sultan A, Steven D, Rostock T, et al. Intravenous administration of magnesium and potassium solution lowers energy levels and increases success rates electrically cardioverting AF. J Cardiovasc Electrophysiol.2012;23 (1):54-9.

16. Shah SA, Clyne CA, Henyan N, et.al. The impact of magnesium sulfate on serum magnesium concentrations and intracellular electrolyte concentrations among patients undergoing radiofrequency catheter ablation. Conn Med 2008;72:261–265.

17. McBride BF, Min B, Kluger J, et al: An evaluation of the impact of oral magnesium lactate on the corrected QT interval of patients receiving sotalol or dofetilide to prevent atrial or ventricular tachyarrhythmia recurrence. Ann Noninv Electro Cardiol 2006; 11:163–9.

18. Dogteroma P, Fua C, Legga T, Chioua Y, et.al.The absolute bioavailability and the effect of food on a new magnesium lactate dihydrate

extended-release caplet in healthy subjects. Drug Dev Ind Pharm. 2018, 44:1481-1487.

19. Kotecha D. Magnesium for AF, Myth or Magic? Circ Arrhythm Electrophysiol. 2016;9: e004521.

20. Elin RJ. Magnesium metabolism in health and disease. Dis Mon. 1988; 34 : 161-218.

21. Rasmussen HS, Thomsen PE. The electrophysiological effects of intravenous magnesium on human sinus node, atrioventricular node, atrium, and ventricle. Clin Cardiol. 1989;12(2):85-90.

22. Avioli L, Berman M. Mg28 kinetics in man. Journal of Applied Physiology.1966; 21:1688-1694.

23. Sun Y, Zhang K, Yu B , et.al. Sweetened Beverages, Genetic Susceptibility, and Incident AF: A Prospective Cohort Study. Circ Arrhythm Electrophysiol. 2024;17:e012145.

24. Zghoul N, Alam-Eldin N, Mak IT, et al. Hypomagnesemia in diabetes patients: comparison of serum and intracellular measurement of responses to magnesium supplementation and its role in inflammation. Diabetes, Metabolic Syndrome, and Obesity: Targets and Therapy. 2018; 11: 1-12.

25. Zhang X, Gobbo, LCD, Hruby A, et.al. The Circulating Concentration and 24-h Urine Excretion of Magnesium Dose- and Time- Dependently Respond to Oral Magnesium

Supplementation in a Meta-Analysis of Randomized Controlled Trials. J Nutra. 2016; 146: 595-602.

26. Coudray C, Rameau M, Feillet-Coudray C, et.al. Study of magnesium bioavailability from ten organic and inorganic Mg salts in Mg-depleted rats using a stable isotope approach. Magnes Res. 2005; 18 (4): 215-23.

27. Graber F; Bioavailability of US Commercial magnesium preparations, Magnes Res. 2001;14: 257-62.

28. Baker WL. Treating arrhythmias with adjunctive magnesium: identifying future research directions. Eur Heart J Cardiovasc Pharmacother. 2017; 3 :108-117.

29. Ranade VV, Somberg JC. Bioavailability and pharmacokinetics of magnesium after administration of magnesium salts to humans. Amer J Ther.2001; 8:345-357.

30. Spencer H, Norris C, Williams D. Inhibitory effects of zinc on magnesium balance and magnesium absorption. J Am Coll Nutr. 1994;13: 479-84.

31. Fine FD, Santa Ana CA, Porter JL, et.al. Intestinal Absorption of Magnesium from Food and Supplements. J Clin Invest. 1991; 88: 396-402.

32. Tohme J, Sleilaty G, Jabbour K, et.al. preoperative oral magnesium loading to prevent

postoperative atrial fibrillation following coronary surgery: a prospective randomized controlled trial. Eur J Cardiothorac Surg. 2022:62: 1-8.

33. Lutsey PL, Chen LY, Eaton A, et.al. A pilot randomized trial of oral magnesium supplementation on supraventricular arrhythmias. Nutrients. 2018; 10: 884.

34. Frick M, Darpo B, Ostergren L, Rosenqvist M. The effect of oral magnesium alone or as an adjuvant to sotalol after cardioversion in patients with persistent atrial fibrillation. Eur Heart J. 2000; 21: 1177-1185.

35. Haigney MCP, Silver B, Tanglao, E, et al. Noninvasive measurement of tissue magnesium and correlation with cardiac levels. Circulation.1995; 92: 2190-2197.

36. Kim SH, Lim KR,Seo JH et.al. Higher heart rate variability as a predictor of AF in patients with hypertension. Sci Rep.2022; 12: 3702.

37. Seaborn GEJ, Todd K, Michael KA, et.al. Heart Rate Variability and Procedural Outcome in Catheter Ablation for AF. Ann Noninvasive Electrocardiol 2014;19(1):23–33.

38. Broux B, De Clercq A., Decloedt A. Heart rate variability parameters in horses distinguish AF from sinus rhythm before and after successful electrical cardioversion. Equine Vet 2017; 49: 723-728.

39. Caron MF, Kluger J, Tsikouris JP, et.al. Effects of intravenous magnesium sulfate on the QT interval in patients receiving Ibutilide. Pharmacology.2003; 23: 296-300.

40. Kalus JS, Spencer AP, Tsikouris JP et.al.Impact of prophylactic i.v. magnesium on the efficacy of ibutilide for conversion of atrial fibrillation or flutter. Am. J Health-Syst Pharm.2002; 60:2308-2312.

41. Robinson CM, Frank FEK. Magnesium lactate in the treatment of Gitelman Syndrome: patient-reported outcomes. Nephrol Dia Transplant. 2016; 0 : 1-5.

42. Baker WL, Kluger J, Coleman CI, White CM. Impact of magnesium-lactate on occurrence of ventricular arrhythmias in patients with implantable cardioverter defibrillators: a randomized, placebo-controlled trial. Open CardiovascMed J 2015;9:83–88.

43. Dobre D, Heijman J, Hiram R et.al. Inflammatory signaling in atrial cardiomyocytes: a novel unifying principle in atrial fibrillation pathophysiology. Nat Rev Cardiol. 2023; 20: 145-167.

44. Kreydiyyeha S I, Abou-Chahinea C, Hilal-Dandanb Interleukin-1β inhibits Na/K ATPase activity and protein expression in cardiac myocytes. Cytokine 26 (2004) 1e8.

45. Niskala A, Heijman J, Dobrev D, Jespersen T, Saljic A. Targeting the NLRP-3 inflammasome

signaling for the management of atrial inflammation. Br J Pharmacol.2024;181:4939-4957.

46. Parks AL, Kim DH, Ko D et.al. Management of atrial fibrillation in older adults. BMJ. 2024; 386: e076246.

47. Hoffman HM, Wright FA, Broide DH, Wanderer AA, Kolodner RD: Identification of a Locus on Chromosome 1q44 for Familial Cold Urticaria. Am J. Hum. Genet. 2000, 66:1693-8.

48. Verma A, Haines DE, Boersma LV et.al. Pulsed Field Ablation for the Treatment of AF: PULSED AFIB Pivotal Trial. Circulation. 2023; 147: 1422-1432.

49. Hindricks G, Potpara T, Dagres N. et al; ESC Scientific Document Group. 2020 ESC Guidelines for the diagnosis and management of AF developed in collaboration with the European Association for Cardio-Thoracic Surgery (EACTS): the task force for the diagnosis and management of AF of the European Society of Cardiology (ESC) developed with the special contribution of the European Heart Rhythm Association (EHRA) of the ESC. Eur Heart J. 2021;42:373–498.

Acknowledgments:

I want to thank my wife, Patricia for her diligent editing of this book; Jennifer Wanderer for the cover graphics (jw@jenniferwanderer.com); Kaitlyn Batzloff Smith and Alan J Zetzer for organizing charts and graphing my data; for helpful commentary from Richard Asarch, M.D.(Mohs surgeon and dermatologist), Eric Weber, M.D.(radiation oncologist), Bart Troy, M.D. (cardiologist), Ron Chin, M.D., (cardiologist), Charles Kirkpatrick, M.D.(Professor of Medicine University of Colorado School of Medicine), Henry Shinefield, M.D.(physician-scientist, infectious disease specialist and a very important mentor); and for the statistical analysis by Kenny Flagg, Ph.D. (flagg.ka@gmail.com).

Also, by Alan A. Wanderer, M.D.

Anaphylaxis, A Medical Thriller

Paperback, e-book, and recently an audiobook*

*Available on all platforms by title, but on Audible it can be accessed only by the author's name.

www.ingramcontent.com/pod-product-compliance
Lightning Source LLC
Chambersburg PA
CBHW050634160426
43194CB00010B/1663